the beauty c

the beauty chronicles

TINA PARSONS

*The Beauty Chronicles is dedicated to my
mother Renate, my daughter Alexa and
my granddaughter Lola who between them
encapsulate the true and lasting essence of beauty*

Praise

"Tina Parsons is one of the most respected people in the beauty world and Habia was delighted when Tina shared her knowledge and experience on our standards development workshops. Tina is a passionate member of the Habia Beauty Forum, giving advice and sharing her knowledge for the benefit of the beauty and holistic industry. Tina has poured her skills into educating hundreds of beauty therapists, many of who have gone on to set up their own salons."

Habia, the industry authority for hair, beauty, nails and spa

"Tina never judges and shows great interest in people in their background, their life and their concerns; she is a true confidante. I have been proud to call her my teacher and I am proud to call her my friend."

Elizabeth Kirby, Holistic Beauty Therapist

"Tina is an inspirational person with extensive knowledge and experience. Her passion for the beauty industry and compassion for her students is outstanding. I feel honoured to have been trained by Tina Parsons."

Jeni Sharpe, Therapist/Recruitment Specialist for the Beauty Industry

"Tina is truly dedicated to the beauty industry. Her knowledge and professionalism is outstanding. With her understanding and experience she is an inspiration to those who meet her. I and fellow beauty therapists who have been trained or worked with Tina are inspired and her knowledge, professionalism and confidence is excellent."

Nicole Palmer-Dimmock

"Tina has the ability to use analogies to make complex subject matters become clear. On a practical level, Tina encourages attention to detail whilst also using gentle insistence on professionalism."

Jan Wasling, Close Health & Beauty

"Tina's depth of knowledge, her professionalism and caring approach for all clients, students and teachers have helped her to achieve so much in the beauty industry. Tina has given me a real buzz for teaching, huge support and mentoring through both my teaching and assessing qualifications. As many have said to me, she is a real inspiration, bringing the best out in everyone."

Jess Dovaston, Beauty therapy lecturer and assessor

"Tina's passion for teaching certainly comes through in all her lessons and during my time as one of her students I suddenly found she had awoken an interest and desire in me to learn more, something I had never felt in my earlier educational years; a truly amazing woman!"

Samantha Hiseman, Equilibrium

"Tina and Decleor have enjoyed a strong and loyal partnership or many years. Tina always demonstrates great dedication and commitment to developing therapists through her training and we are privileged to work so closely with such an industry professional. With Tina's holistic approach and calming influences her advice and direction within the beauty industry is unparalleled."

Martine Archer, Decleor and Carita UK

"Tina has given me guidance throughout my professional life. I have looked to her for advice on many things, from professionalism and updating my skills and qualifications to concerns within my job role and with beauty and holistic therapies. Her pursuit of knowledge and her insistence on high standards are inspirational."

Pam Reed, Beauty and holistic therapy assessor and verifier

"Tina was an excellent teacher, always very professional and supportive on all levels. She was very helpful when I was starting my business with regard to general business advice as well as more practical issues. She always has been, and still is, a great source of information and support for me."

Jayne Reading, Pure

Acknowledgements

My thanks go to colleagues, clients, students and friends who have collectively inspired, encouraged, motivated and supported me in the writing of this book. To my family, especially my daughter Alexa and husband Chris, I extend my heartfelt thanks and love for their unwavering belief in me. I would also like to thank the team at Bookshaker for turning my vision into a reality.

Foreword

It is incredibly exciting, and indeed a privilege, to be asked to write the foreword for *The Beauty Chronicles*, not only because I feel honoured to be chosen to do so, but because it relates to my industry, which I have been a major part of for over 40 years.

I was there during the early years of the beauty industry and have been a passionate contributor to how it has evolved, specifically educationally, into the major entity it has become today.

I was first introduced to Tina Parsons when I visited her newly established private training centre (in Peterborough). My role at that time was to advise her on implementing the necessary courses which would help it to become the highly acclaimed centre it is today.

Tina herself is one of the hardest working therapists I have had the privilege of meeting. She never tires of supporting the industry at all levels, including advising the Skills Sector bodies in creating and updating standards for training, thereby assuring qualifications are managed in line with current industry trends. This is such an important factor and one which I know all dedicated professionals in our industry are keen to ensure are followed through.

Over the years I have witnessed Tina go from strength to strength; she has written many books to support therapists, enabling them to progress swiftly and efficiently through their development.

It is wonderful to see how she has now adapted her guidance into a book which can help everyone, not just those in the industry. It is informative as well as thought-provoking.

I have every intention of continuing to strive for the best in the beauty industry for many years to come, but it is truly wonderful and satisfying to see others, like Tina, grow and take the mantle forward into the future.

Gerri Moore
Vice-President of FHT (Federation of Holistic Therapists)
and Chief Verifier for VTCT

Contents

Introduction

Charms strike the sight, but merit wins the soul.

Alexander Pope

Beauty: the impressions associated with all that can be experienced through the human senses and the combination of the qualities and circumstances that produce them.

For me beauty began as far back as I can remember. Romantic images of the late 1950s glamour as my parents and their friends attended parties and balls in the officer's mess in Singapore will stay forever in my mind. The bright, shiny painted faces and nails of the women were something that stood out most especially for me and they were something that I longed for more than anything else throughout my childhood years and as I was forbidden to wear make-up or nail enamel until my mid teens I all but counted the days until then.

By the 1960s we were living in forces Germany and I experienced the swinging sixties of England second hand via the growing media of the day, I drooled over the fashion and beauty colour photographs in my *Jackie* magazine each week, waited with bated breath for parcels from my grandmother in England, with the latest makeup products from Rimmel, and sat glued to my seat at the Saturday morning cinema to catch

1

sight of Twiggy, the Beatles et al on the newsreels. I built my own fantasy world based around my limited exposure and knowledge of the world at that time and this fed my growing passion, fuelled my ambition and sealed my fate. It was then that I decided that the world of beauty was for me.

Returning to rural England in the early seventies, my image of the beauty world took a turn for the worse. Everywhere was dull and grey; I could not find the bright colours of my eye shadow palettes or the glamour of my teen magazines on the streets of my new hometown and where, oh where were the beautiful young people in their patterned miniskirts and bright mini cars? I felt cheated and betrayed, unaware that things were to get duller and greyer as the coal miners' strikes led to the three-day week and doom and gloom in all senses of the word.

As my school days came to an end I needed to find my world of beauty more than ever. Career advisers at school sneered at my quest for beauty, implying that it was a fickle and unsuitable world. Instead they suggested that I and indeed every other girl in our school train to become a secretary, nurse or teacher.

I refused to believe that the world I dreamt of did not exist, but I compromised.

I embarked on a two-year full time hairdressing course at the local college at the age of 16, thus keeping my teachers and parents happy as I secured an all important (in their eyes) trade, albeit still slightly unsuitable and certainly not as suitable as becoming a secretary, nurse or teacher, but as I had been willing to compromise I guess they felt obliged to also.

An advert in a glossy magazine in the hair salon where I worked as a Saturday girl initiated my eventual and inevitable move into the professional world of beauty.

I became an Innoxa Girl in 1974 in beautiful Bond Street, home of the infamous beauty salons. Next to Vidal Sassoon's flagship hairdressers, and above the renowned Innoxa beauty salon, the Innoxa School for Beauty Therapy and Beauty Culture looked out onto all that was glamorous, expensive and exclusive in 1970s London.

It was one of only a handful of schools to offer beauty training in the UK at that time and the answer to my hopes and dreams.

Our rivals were the girls from the Lucie Clayton Grooming School, (a popular finishing school of the day) who occupied rooms on the opposite side of the street. Whilst they were busy finishing we were busy starting.

We felt we had the edge – modern girls embarking on a career that had the potential to take us further than the arms of a husband.

I was suddenly thrust into the real life world of the cinema newsreels and on to the pages of my magazines.

London was all I had imagined the world of beauty to be and whilst I remained on the periphery for much of the time, with neither the money nor the courage to truly take part, I was an avid observer and revelled in all I saw.

The bright visions of my imagination were there in Technicolour in the many faces of beauty as hippy flowers turned to punk passion and new romantic highwaymen and women, interspersed with traditional Sloane Rangers. 1970s London was a melting pot of beauty, spewing out different images of itself at every moment. The tube stations, the buses, the streets, the shops, the pubs and clubs all thronged with a vibrancy that can still be seen and felt today.

My new world not only contained the glamour of my childhood memories and the promise of my teenage imagination, but one that would ultimately take me on a lifetime's journey into the realms of beauty. This had many twists and turns along the way as my arrival coincided with one of the busiest times in the history of the beauty industry. Whilst the modern world was testing beauty boundaries, with the stars of the day advertising the latest products and innovations, we Innoxa girls in our pristine white uniforms, with makeup-perfect complexions and not a hair out of place, represented the secret face of the beauty industry; we learnt professional skills that had until now been accessible only to the privileged wealthy.

All this exclusivity was about to change.

Some of the developments that have occurred since the 1970s are worth celebrating: as we apply a product to our bodies we can now be assured that it does what it says on the package, and know that it will do us more good than harm.

But we should also be aware of the facts and theories gained along the way and become more responsible for their use and accountable for their abuse.

Beauty is both a science and an art. Once we accept this, it may be possible to determine if beauty can be found in a tub or tube, achieved with a brush and palette, acquired under a needle or knife, applied as a spritz or spray or taken as a potion or pill, and thus balance the fantasy of a beautiful image with the reality of true beauty.

In *The Beauty Chronicles* I have tried to answer these questions and unravel the origins and developments of some of our best kept beauty secrets, as well as question where today's controversial and contradictory beauty industry is leading us.

Tina Parsons

Introduction

CHAPTER ONE

Perception

Breasts and bottoms look boringly alike.
Faces, though, can be quite different and
a damn sight more interesting!
Lee Remick

Perception could be described as our ultimate sensation. It is formed in the brain through the processing of sight, touch, smell, taste and sound. Perception is the ultimate experience of our world and is our final judge of beauty.

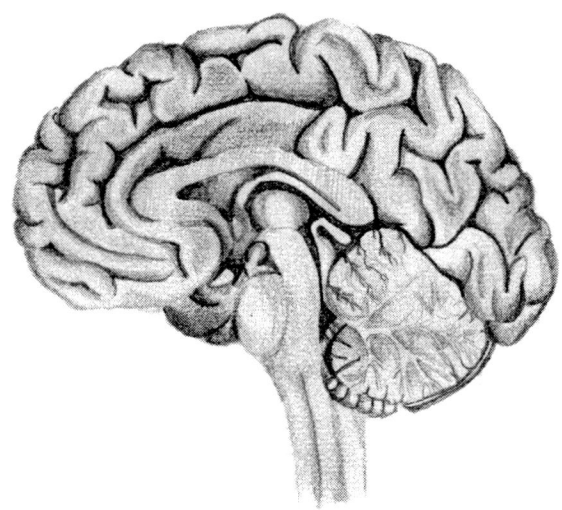

PERCEPTION

The term beauty in English comes from the French *beauté*, derived from the Latin *bellus*, which in its feminine form is *bella* and refers to something that is pleasing to see, feel, hear, smell or taste.

Beauty is involved in every one of our senses, helps to form the basis of our memories and provides us with a unique set of standards with which to view the world and be viewed in return.

The brain analyses the sensations it receives from the sensory organs of the eyes, skin, nose, mouth, and ears. The resulting information is added to and compared with that already in the brain's memory bank and a verdict is produced. It is this verdict that forms a person's perception of beauty and is responsible for the associated emotional response.

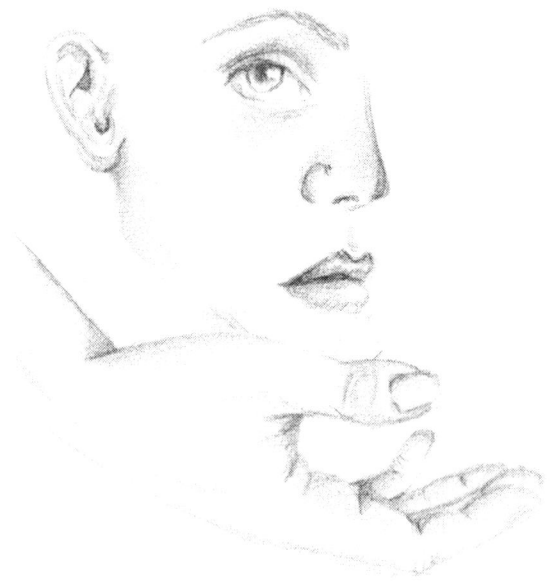

THE SPECIAL SENSES

The Science of the Senses

The central nervous system consists of the **brain** and **spinal cord** which are responsible for controlling the body. Radiating out from the brain and spinal cord are the **peripheral nerves** – 12 pairs from the brain and 31 pairs from the spinal cord.

These nerves supply the body with the ability to sense a stimulus and act upon it by sending messages in the form of electrical impulses to and from the brain via **sensory** and **motor nerves.**

The cranial nerves are arranged from 1-12 as follows:

- **Olfactory** – associated with our sense of smell
- **Optic** – associated with our sense of sight
- **Oculomotor** – associated with the movement of the eyes
- **Trochlear** – assist with the movement of the eyes
- **Trigeminal** – associated with activity in the eyes and jaw
- **Abducent** – help with eye movements
- **Facial** – associated with the sense of taste, production of saliva and tears and contribute to controlling facial expressions
- **Vestibulocochlear** – associated with the ears and help with our sense of balance and hearing

- **Glossopharyngeal** – associated with the tongue, the throat and help to control swallowing
- **Vagus** – associated with the action of the mouth in terms of speech and swallowing as well as being associated with heart, thorax and abdomen
- **Accessory** – associated with the back and neck
- **Hypoglossal** – associated with speaking, chewing and swallowing

The 31 pairs of spinal nerves form networks or groups from which they divide and branch out to provide all parts of the body with the ability to feel and respond.

The **central nervous system** together with the peripheral nerves forms both an internal and external communication system that receives and integrates data from the sensory organs. This initiates a sensorial emotion in response to the forces of the ever-changing face of beauty to which it is constantly being exposed.

The Art of the Senses

In addition to the coming together of the physical senses and the emotional links associated with sight, touch, sound, smell and taste in what we know as perception, some believe in the potential for joining this with information gained by other, less quantifiable means and resulting in "extra sensory perception".

Whilst the physical and emotional aspects of the sensory organs rely on the energy produced in the body via the nervous system, the "extra sensory" functions rely on a type of energy that is harder to define yet equally powerful, gaining its strength from spirituality rather than physicality.

No word exists in the English language to describe this type of energy but in Eastern cultures it is referred to as *chi* (Chinese), *ki* (Japanese) and *prana* (Sanskrit) where the belief systems subscribe to the idea that this energy links the earth with the universe and has the power to affect and be affected by everything of the past, present and future.

Like the energy of the nervous system, this type of energy flows around and through the body, but unlike physical energy it flows through channels that as yet have not been scientifically proven. Light is said to carry this energy and its channels within the body are known as auras, meridians, zones and chakras.

An **aura** describes the energy channel that surrounds a living being and is made up of seven bodies or layers which link the physical, emotional and spiritual aspects of life.

The **meridian system** describes one key channel for energy within the body that divides into 14 major branches. Each branch is known as a meridian. Twelve meridians are linked to specific organs within the body and the remaining two regulate the energy flow into and out of the body as a whole.

Zone theory refers to the concept of the body being linked through 10 longitudinal channels that run parallel to one another, from the tip of the thumbs/fingers through the body to the tip of the toes. Each zone provides a pathway for energy flow.

The **chakra system** refers to energy channels that provide the ultimate link between the external and internal energies of the body. Often referred to as wheels of light, the chakras form seven main centres along the central longitudinal line, radiating out to affect all parts of the body. Energy is able to enter and exit the body via the chakras, creating an indelible link.

The energy that flows within these various channels remains elusive and difficult to detect by the physical senses alone and requires the extra sensory functions to determine its value in the form of:

- **Clairvoyance** – clear vision
- **Clairsentience** – clear feeling
- **Clairalience** – clear smelling
- **Clairgustance** – clear taste
- **Clairaudience** – clear hearing

The combined forces of these result in **claircognisance** or **clear knowing,** which describes the ultimate extra sensory function associated with perception, adding another dimension to the judgment of beauty. Under such scrutiny, beauty becomes multi-faceted, with each physical, emotional and spiritual sensory function providing the means to investigate all of its many layers in a quest to find its intimate truth.

What is Beauty?

Every generation and era has believed that it held the key to beauty. No trip to a museum or stately home, or leaf through an historical novel or biography takes place without finding some reference to the beautification of the men and women of the time.

The fascination with historical evidence of human vanity and the accompanying beauty ideals it provokes is strong and influences each generation to evolve their own style of beauty.

Beauty, at its best, enables a person to develop a sense of identity, well-being and belonging. At its worst, however, beauty is responsible for self-destruction, mutilation and isolation.

Each new culture and generation believes that theirs is true beauty when what they are actually peddling is far from the truth – or is it? The Emperor's New Clothes?

There can be no ultimate definition of beauty; different cultures throughout history have held and continue to hold differing and often conflicting views and ideals.

How many white skinned people view their milky complexions with disgust as they strive for the all over tan associated with sun beds, sprays and creams whilst their darker skinned counterparts use a whole host of tried and not always well tested means to lighten their skins?

Pride as well as prejudice has a lot to answer for in the quest for skin colour. Historically the lighter skinned people of the world showed off their wealth through foreign travel of which a tan was the living proof, whilst those with darker skins, keen to demonstrate that their wealth meant they no longer worked out of doors, were able to hold their heads up higher as their skin lightened.

Theorists have laboured long and hard, coming up with complicated even mathematical explanations that feed our enquiring minds with left-brain logic. Popular theories are based on ideas associated with beauty for survival of the species and studies have gone a long way to prove that there are certain ideals that cross cultural boundaries.

The main reason for this is rooted in sexual selection. Post puberty the ideal male and female bodies take on the form of that which is most suited to reproduction. The secondary sexual characteristics associated with a person's move from childhood to adulthood become the basis of sexual attraction: the male becomes more muscular and strong and the female more curvaceous and soft. As a result of these differences, at a basic level, they become more attractive to one another.

The survival of the fittest relies on strong levels of immunity, which have been proved to be associated with those male and female adults who take on the most ideal post pubescent physical forms.

Additional theories subscribe to the notion that symmetry can explain the links between what we find attractive and thus beautiful and what we don't and that these theories are universal.

One such theory is based on the golden proportions of ancient Greece – a set of mathematical equations whereby the face and body can be measured against an ideal e.g. the ideal waist to hip ratio of approximately 0.70 accurately indicates most women's fertility.

> To calculate a female's waist to hip ratio:
> 1. Measure the waist at the narrowest part
> 2. Measure the hips around the widest part of the buttocks
> 3. Divide the waist measurement by the hip measurement

More recent theories of symmetry have looked not so much at proportions but more at the similarities between the left and right sides of the body. Scientific evidence supports this ideal as not only being universal but also crossing the boundaries of age.

Babies are reported to spend more time staring at pictures of faces that are symmetrical. The faces and bodies of the most photographed people of the world have either a greater natural symmetry than average or, more often, have had that symmetry reproduced by cosmetic and/or digital enhancement. Research has also shown that not only does symmetry result in a higher mate value and stronger levels of immunity, but also greater success in other areas of life including education and work, career development, personal success and ultimately quality of life. This in turn has helped to make the beauty industry a global - and continuously lucrative - phenomenon.

But the focus on the physicality of beauty remains one-sided with explanations that quench the thirst for knowledge associated with a linear mode of thinking and our need for left-brain analysis and explanation. When it comes to scientific research the oft forgotten and lesser-used right-brain circular mode of thinking associated with creativity and intuition, whereby the potential to synthesise rather than analyse the facts surrounding beauty ideals has less of a focus.

Whilst outer physical perfection has the potential to provide us with an instant beauty fix with its associated feel good factor, a person's inner beauty may be harder to perceive and define.

Many males as well as females will list a sense of humour, intelligence, congeniality, integrity, kindness and empathy as providing the beauty behind the twinkle in the eye, capable of initiating the spark of mutual attraction on all levels.

Once this level of attraction has been reached, the physical attributes fade in importance as inner beauty complements and compensates for their outer appearance.

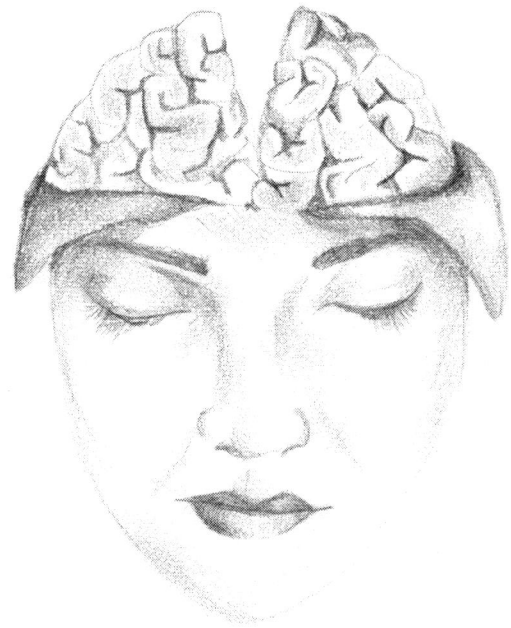

RIGHT BRAIN/LEFT BRAIN

Right = creativity. Enjoys mystery and ambiguity – capable of intuitive thought

Left = logic. Enjoys clarity and can formulate specific and rational thoughts

Perhaps herein lies the key to perception of what is truly beautiful. It may also make sense of perceptions of the changing faces of beauty throughout a person's lifetime. This has potential to achieve a greater balanced outlook for the future of human beauty and dispel the spiralling myths that have accompanied its long and troublesome development.

Beauty for Power and Attraction

Beauty in its many guises is used as a tool to empower its holder and attract the beholder. The tattooing, scarring, piercing and painting of the face and body together with the application of chemicals, electrical currents and surgery by different cultures worldwide have long been associated with enhancement, alteration, correction, preservation, maintenance, improvement and recreation.

This power of attraction formed the basis for the early standards of beauty. Inspiration was sought in nature as observation of the natural magnetism of all that was best in the animal and plant kingdoms proved that beauty did indeed hold the key to the human need to find a mate and aspire to and achieve greatness.

Primitive forms of make-up were artistically applied. People imagined they took on the characteristics of the wildlife they imitated by adopting cat-like eyes, tiger-striped bodies and plant style faces and bodies Mystical symbols of the sun, moon and stars drew attention to parts of the body to emulate the beauty and power of the universe or in the 17th/18th century , to disguise imperfections.

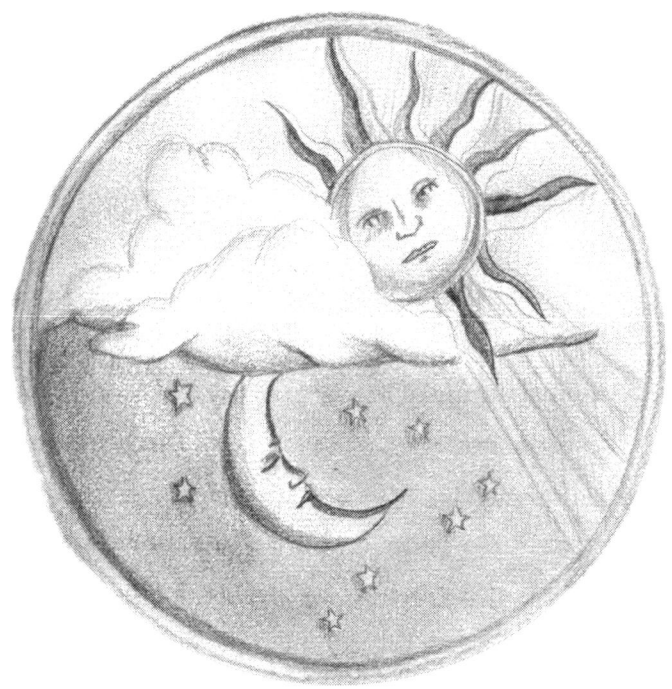

Inspired by nature, colour became an important tool, and remains so today. Face and body makeup was often made with toxic ingredients, unfortunately, so experimentation did not always have a happy ending! Heroes and heroines of each era had a powerful influence. From Cleopatra to Princess Diana, from Bette Davis to Madonna, from geishas to suffragettes, from the courtesans of the past to the super models of today, these heroines have all contributed to shifts in the perception of beauty.

What Goes Around Comes Around

Familiarity breeds contempt - each new generation looks to find another influence upon which to base their beauty ideal and the world of beauty swings between the understated and the excessive.

Politics and religion have both altered the perception of beauty over the ages. The boom in the mid to late 20th century caused the use of beauty products and makeup to soar as the developed world found beauty in all that was excessive, bright and colourful.

Conversely, the puritanical Victorians turned away from the cosmetics, colour and strong aromas that had proved so popular in Elizabethan times towards all that was pure, clean and natural.

We are now moving into a time where technology rules. Education and knowledge is greater than it has ever been but we remain only a click away from the past. There are many lessons in beauty to be learned from the past and choices to be made for the future. Are we ready to take responsibility and recognize our mistakes and learn from them?

Beauty for Seduction, Selection and Survival

Everyone is looking for a kindred spirit and a suitable mate to ensure the survival of their species.

We are drawn to what we think is beautiful, and choose the mate that conforms to our taste, which in turn leads to seduction and ultimately the survival of the species. Beauty is comfortable in many guises.

The recognition parents and grandparents have for their young results in the beauty of unconditional love.

A baby responds to and reflects the beauty it recognises in its primary carers, developing an unbreakable bond through a set of mutual and exclusive positive facial expressions, pet words and deeds resulting in memories that bind for a lifetime.

A child is drawn like a magnet to the beauty it intuitively recognises in another, most often found in the same sex, with whom firm friendships naturally develop that are without judgment or prejudice.

A young adult possesses and is attracted to the beauty of a suitable mate - although they may need to keep trying before they make their final decision.

From ageing originality emerges and the beauty that results from life experiences and beginning to know oneself. This has the potential for a deeper insight and understanding of the multifaceted face of beauty.

At its best beauty equals or inspires love and all that is natural, real and honest. Its darker side, however, has as its foundations much that is fake, synthetic and unnatural. One side cannot exist without the other and therein lies a state of balance and harmony reflecting the diversity which offers a true reflection of beauty.

However, there is a flaw. Vanity is an example of pride and narcissism, which in Christian teachings is one of the seven deadly sins along with envy, gluttony, lust, anger, greed and sloth. Vanity causes people to crave and aim for a superficial beauty, often unrealistic, unattainable and thus impossible to maintain. It also causes people to concentrate on their appearance to the detriment of other, less apparent beauty.

> Narcissism is the term given to a condition characterised by excessive admiration of oneself. In Greek mythology Narcissus was a beautiful hunter who died from the love of his own beauty once he had seen it reflected in a pool of water. He changed into a flower bearing the same name. Narcissi are bulbous flowering plants including the daffodil.

Narcissism in the young is often accompanied by anxiety with their developing bodies whilst trying to adapt to current fashions in order to conform. Older people have their own vanity issues most commonly with aging, as they fail to recognise the beauty of originality in the middle and latter stages of life and try to recapture the beauty of their past.

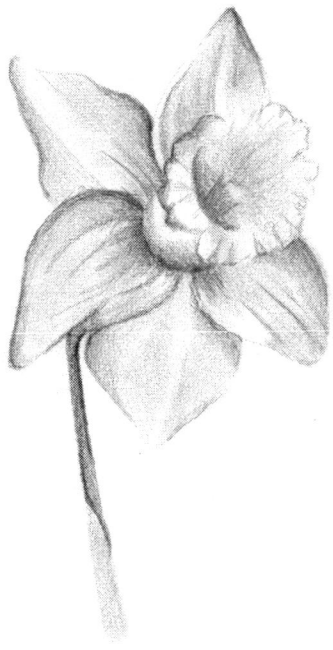

NARCISSUS

Vanity can result in a false beauty identity that may conflict with a person's true beauty, affecting the way in which they are viewed by others as well as how they live and enjoy their lives. The confusion that often accompanies the various stages or cycles of life may have as much to do with nature as it does with nurture.

The beauty standards of each generation are as fickle as they are fashionable. Our superficial beauty ideals change with the season, the era and the influences put upon us.

At a deeper level however, nature has equipped us to deal with the cycles of life as the electrical and chemical reactions associated with our development are activated and the relevant directives acted out as per instructions i.e.

- Childhood growth and development
- Puberty and fertility
- Pregnancy and reproduction
- Female menopause and male equivalent, andropause

New life is formed from the production, reproduction and interaction of billions of individual cells. Each cell has an individual life span and collectively they have specific functions to fulfil. The interaction between the cells is paramount to maintain a fully functioning human physically, psychologically and spiritually.

Physical

The cells of the physical body form its basic structure and function by grouping together as body systems:

- The **integumentary** system: the skin, hair and nails performing the functions associated with protection of the body
- The **skeletal** system: a framework of bones and joints that support the physical body
- The **muscular** system: providing the body with a range of voluntary and involuntary muscles for internal and external movement

- The **respiratory** system: processing the body's oxygen through the airways and lungs
- The **circulatory** systems: a network of transportation vessels leading to and away from the heart
- The **digestive** system: processing the nutrients needed to sustain the life of the body through ingestion (mouth), digestion (stomach), absorption (small intestines) and elimination (large intestine)
- The **urinary** system: filtering the blood of cellular waste and unwanted substances through the production, storage, and elimination of urine via the kidneys, bladder and urethra
- The **immune** system: the body's resistance to and defence from that which may cause harm
- The **nervous** system: a means of communication within the whole body through the production of electrical impulses that link the body with brain and spinal chord
- The **endocrine** system: a chemical means of internal body communication via the production of hormones by specific, strategically placed glands

Psychological

The activity within the brain that is responsible for reacting with reality and producing a sense of individuality in the form of:

- **Ego:** that which is devoted to 'I' and the sense of self in relation to the social standards of the day
- **Id:** that which is associated with the inherited instinctive impulses of an individual as part of the unconscious
- **Psyche:** that which is considered apart from the body

Spiritual

Connected with the inner life and being of a person in the form of:

- **Soul:** the immaterial part of a living being which thinks and wills and may be regarded by some as being immortal
- **Spirit:** the vital animating essence of a living being containing the life-giving principle

A complex balancing act between the physical, psychological and spiritual energy accompanies a human being throughout life and exists through the series of life cycles that control every aspect of a person's development in both the short and long term.

History has shown that the distance between the cycles is ever decreasing and the need to change the next cycle ever increasing. Beauty boundaries are regularly broken as the young are encouraged to appear ever older and the ageing ever younger. The desire to conform is very stressful and a state of confusion sets in.

Walk the Walk and Talk the Talk

The way in which a person lives, thinks and acts has a constant effect on maintaining a sense of internal and external balance which ultimately has a knock on effect on beauty.

Ignorance and a lack of self-awareness and understanding often results in imbalance as a person experiences the effects of what is commonly described as stress. Over time our means of survival have changed and so too has the nature of stress. Stress may be classified as anything that puts the body into a state of action and nowadays it is not so much associated with 'fight or flight' but more with 'struggle and strife'. Stress, like beauty comes in a variety of guises, which may be personal or general, physical, psychological and even spiritual and initiates a set of reactions within the body designed to cope well in the short term but can lead to destruction and decay if not counteracted in the long term.

A stressor is detected by the body via the sensory organs, which in turn alert the brain to produce a set of chemical messengers or hormones to help deal with the impending danger. Two such hormones are cortisol and adrenalin.

Cortisol helps the body maintain a resistance to stress while adrenalin activates the body to deal with the stressor by initiating the following reactions within the body:

- Increased levels of **breathing** to improve oxygen levels
- Increased **blood flow to the brain** to improve mental activity
- Increased **blood flow to the muscles** to improve muscle strength and endurance
- Increased **vision** as the pupils dilate
- Increased **sweating** to reduce body temperature
- Increased **power** as the liver releases its energy store
- **Reduced blood flow** to digestive and urinary organs

Stress may have a warrior/worrier effect by producing in a person the physical strength to attack the stressor or the mental power to worry about it and may be seen as being constructive or destructive and as such safe *and* unsafe.

Safe stress enables the body to function at its optimum levels. It provides the impetus to get motivated, to be optimistic and to achieve against adversity. It may be seen as the means to following a dream, felt as a driving force and heard as a little voice within providing a means for inner encouragement and guidance. It may be associated with the X factor that makes us stand out from the crowd.

Such stress has the power to promote positive action but as with all power it needs to be regularly refuelled and serviced ie replenished through breathing, eating and drinking, sleeping and with positive thoughts and rejuvenated through excretion of waste and the relinquishing of negative thoughts in order to maintain its energy and remain within safe limits for the wellbeing of the whole body.

Unsafe stress occurs when the balance between power and energy is lost, as the signs for refuelling are either not acted upon correctly or ignored completely.

There is excess production of stress hormones, and the body remains in a constant state of 'fight or flight' without the benefit of refuelling and servicing. The natural coping mechanisms of the body start to degenerate. This is known as the General Adaptation Syndrome or GAS, which tracks the course of stress through three distinctive stages.

Stage One – Alarm

An initial stressful situation sets off the release of stress hormones and the body experiences a set of symptoms including:

- **Quick, shallow breathing** as the body attempts to take in more oxygen in order to fuel the body ready for action.
- **Racing heart** in an attempt to pump more oxygen to the muscles.

- Feeling of tummy **butterflies** as blood is diverted away from the digestive organs in favour of the muscles etc.

- **Trembling** eg shaky hands as muscles prepare for action.

- **Hot and clammy hands** as body temperature rises and the skin produces sweat in order to keep cool.

These are all natural reactions to a real or perceived stressor and are intended to alert the body to the possible danger ahead in preparation for action ie 'fight or flight'.

Stage Two – Resistance

As a stressful situation increases, additional pressure is put on the body's coping mechanisms resulting in a set of common symptoms including:

- **Aching muscles** as muscles that were ready for action become overworked

- **Headaches** as mental and physical strain begin to develop

- **Loss of appetite** as digestive organs fail to function properly

- **Difficulty sleeping** as the mind and body are unable to switch off

- **Lethargy** as the body uses up its energy reserve

Not only do these symptoms accompany an increase in stress but they also result in a tendency for a person to become more susceptible to acute conditions such as diarrhoea, frequent colds, thrush and cystitis as the body's natural immunity is weakened.

Stage Three – Exhaustion

Continuous and prolonged stress results in a gradual weakening of the organs and body systems responsible for coping with and resisting stress. The body starts to lose its natural defence mechanisms and cells are unable to regenerate. This stage is associated with chronic and degenerative illness as the body can no longer maintain its state of balance or homeostasis ie migraines, diabetes, high blood pressure. The excessive use and abuse of food, alcohol, drugs, exercise and sex is also associated with this stage as a person clutches at short term relief.

Long term, unsafe stress and the resulting general adaptation syndrome force the body and mind to experience changes resulting in an increased vulnerability which may manifest itself in any of the following:

- **Disease** as immunity is lowered
- **Wear and tear** due to overuse and lack of care
- **Premature ageing** as the body's natural defence is lowered

- **Neurosis** eg anxiety, phobias, obsession and depression as normal thoughts and feelings spiral out of control
- **Psychosis** as in extreme cases a loss of contact with reality may occur

Stress, like vanity presents another flaw in the beauty story as the pressure mounts to conform to a certain kind of image instigated by the Barbie/Sindy doll phenomena of recent years, which is increasingly hard to come by and for many, totally impractical and out of reach

The Barbie/Sindy dolls have become iconic figures the world over and one that many females aspire to regardless of age, race, colour or creed. The look and indeed the feel of these dolls have infiltrated the minds of boys as well as girls in the playground to become considered the ideal female form. The Barbie/Sindy image in reality captures a fleeting moment of a female's life cycle yet she inspires the very young who have not yet reached that moment to speed up the hands of time whilst those who are past the moment go all out to push back time. Stress becomes the by-product as well as the side effect.

A prediction for the future sees stress levels rising and less and less to differentiate the natural cycles of life as they spiral out of control in a quest to alter the hands of time. Will beauty become faceless as its many guises merge into one and time loses its meaning?

Life cycles are like the seasons - spring brings new life, summer sees it bloom and flourish, with autumn comes ripeness and change, and winter a slowing down before a natural end. As climate change merges the seasons unnaturally, will it also bring with it a merging of the life cycles of its people and/or vice versa forcing natural beauty into a false future?

As a result the perception of beauty is laden with contradiction and fraught with confusion, while an industry gets richer and richer.

But where *does* the beauty industry stand in all of this?

On the one hand it has empowered generations of people with the means to achieve beauty through natural enhancement with products and treatments that are increasingly safe to use and effective. On the other, it continues to contribute to the rising stress levels associated with body image, self esteem and confidence by promoting unnatural beauty images through extensive marketing and strong advertising.

The beauty industry as we know it today emerged in the 19th century as a handful of entrepreneurs identified a potential profit in transforming the many small traditional cottage industries associated with health and beauty into global businesses contributing to the world's economy at the highest competitive level. The homemade creams and lotions whose recipes passed down through generations were developed by apothecaries, pharmacists and chemists before being sold to a wider market. Other such products were developed as by-products of those associated with the workplace.

Prior to this time attaining beauty as well as health relied more on luck than judgment. Trial and error accounted for much of the cultural rituals and customs that developed across the world and were associated as much with protection, healing and cleansing as they were with beauty. There was little or no scientific evidence as to their effectiveness, although they were often kept as closely guarded secrets passed down through generations and thus prone to becoming lost or misinterpreted over the passage of time.

> Vaseline is a petroleum derivative which was first used to heal cuts and bruises amongst oil rig workers

All too often the positive or negative reactions of substances (internally consumed or applied externally) were not widely understood and so became associated with underground activity, witchcraft and more often than not linked with immorality, evil and the devil. Fatal mistakes were commonplace as lives were lost to the cause of health and beauty through misuse of harmful substances.

> Drops of the poisonous deadly nightshade plant were frequently used during Elizabethan times to make the pupils appear larger and the eyes brighter. Faces were whitened by many early cultures with a thick layer of toxic, lead-based paint with fatal consequences as a result of long term use.

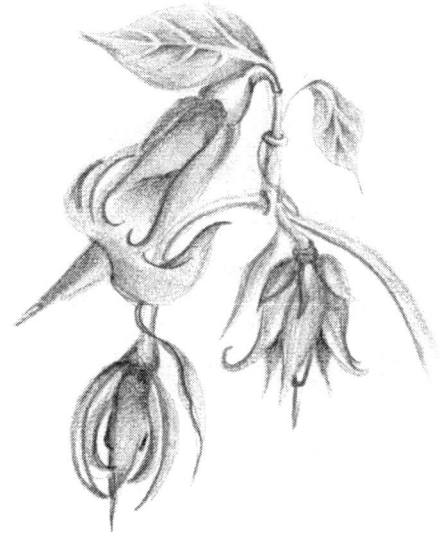

DEADLY NIGHTSHADE

Conversely lives were saved by the use of herbs and spices whose properties were found, often by accident, to be not only healing and curative but also anti -ageing and protective.

> The healing properties of some plants were found quite by accident eg when a French chemist accidentally burnt himself whilst working, he reached for the nearest liquid in which to soak his burn and was amazed by the resulting action. The liquid was lavender oil and the resulting action was a level of healing he had not previously been witness to.

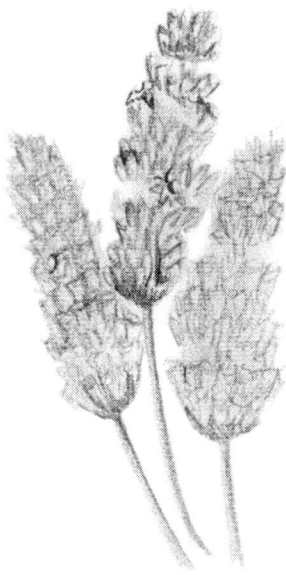

LAVENDER

Health and beauty have always been linked; history demonstrates that traditionally they were very much the domain of royalty but as more people began to travel, the trade in ingredients and knowledge widened to allow the wealthy to get in on the act.

The industrial revolution opened the channels of trade further and products became available to the mass market. Travel also brought with it stories of beauty rituals from far flung places and nowadays we are as comfortable with the ancient art of health and beauty from Eastern cultures as we are with scientific advancements made by the Western world.

Whilst the Western civilisation developed so did knowledge of energy. The development of electricity coincided with the discovery of the electrical impulses that exist within the human body that link the nervous system with the rest of the body systems. This brought about the use of electrical machines to assist the functioning of the body for medical purposes that were later adapted for use in beautifying the body eg the use of high frequency, galvanic, faradic and micro currents for face and body.

Eastern cultures meanwhile continued their voyage of discovery less scientifically working with the natural energy ie chi, ki and prana that was felt to exist within the body as well as circulate around it. Treatments that balanced this energy were developed eg acupuncture, shiatsu and Indian head massage.

However, the mixed messages that accompany the history of health and beauty have also created arguments that continue to rage today. There have been times when cleanliness has been seen as being next to godliness but by the same token the cleansing and bathing rituals that were made popular in ancient Egyptian and Roman times were viewed as immoral and sinful by later generations.

The use of makeup and perfumes to enhance beauty has been a popular ideal over the years but yet has also been viewed as suitable only for ladies of ill repute. Historical evidence also demonstrates the fluctuations in popularity of hairy and non-hairy body parts for both men and women. Massage treatments whilst used extensively by many ancient peoples of the world for their therapeutic benefits were also banned by others because of their associations with sex, sin and debauchery. But whilst time has brought many inconsistencies as to the right or wrong ways to maintain the body, parallels can also be found in the development of health and beauty rituals that were intuitive and experimental and met the basic needs of life. Every culture and tradition developed products to be used on the body dependent on the availability of raw ingredients. Products were sought to cleanse, protect and moisturise the body as well as to prevent and cure illness.

The Egyptians regularly used crocodile excrement in mud baths to firm and tone the skin whilst Cleopatra is purported to have bathed in milk and honey to maintain her complexion. Honey is still used today in many skin care products.

The Romans had a passion for bathing, sweating and massaging, with a variety of scented oils. They claimed almond oil effaced wrinkles and when mixed with honey removed blemishes from the face. Almond oil is still a popular carrier oil used in today's massage treatments.

Combs became popular tools in the early medieval period, used to limit the inconvenience caused by head lice as well as to encourage natural oils from the skin. They also applied oils along the length of hair for shine and condition in much the same way as conditioners are combed through the hair today.

The middle ages saw crude mouthwashes being used to combat the odours resulting from poor dental health and hygiene. Common ingredients were mint and myrrh which when diluted in wine proved effective and refreshing. Herbalists still use myrrh for its antibacterial properties; mint is widely used for its fresh smell and digestive properties whilst alcohol remains a useful preservative.

Many of the larger homes in the 16th/17th century had a still-room where herbs and spices were formulated from traditional recipes into healing remedies, as well as adapted for cosmetic use. Over the centuries, such recipes have been adapted and expanded to meet current health and beauty demands.

Washballs were popular in the 18th century. Bathing was a rare occurrence, but washballs, often blended with whitening agents, were used primarily on the hands for cleansing but perhaps more importantly for the ladies of the day, to beautify them by restoring paleness. Hand washes and whitening creams are popular hand care treatments today.

In some parts of the world, clean water was a luxury and often carried the diseases that repeatedly wiped out whole sections of communities. As a result washing, as we know it today, was not always an option. Bodily waste was removed using leaves or bark and skin was wiped with oils often infused with herbs and spices, hair was powdered to absorb the dirt and grease whilst teeth rotted away as little emphasis was placed on the type of cleanliness that we have become accustomed to today.

There are still those of us who can remember that bathing and hair washing was a weekly ritual, whilst daily showering was non-existent. And only a few years before that, bathrooms had no place within an ordinary household. Toilets were consigned to outhouses, with toilet paper that was rough, hard and lacking in any absorbent properties. Bathtubs were brought out on rare occasions and placed in front of the fire, filled with water for the whole family to take it in turns to bathe in.

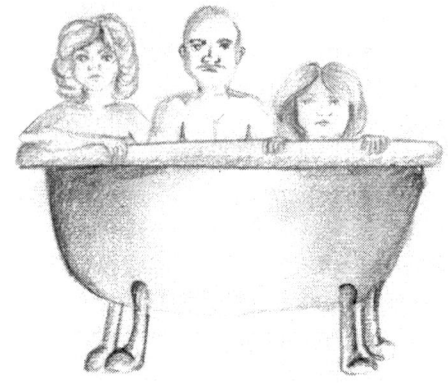

The wealthy used perfumes to wash and freshen their bodies and homes and frequently covered their skins with a whole host of often toxic pastes to hide the imperfections and sores that inevitably developed from poor hygiene.

The gradual advances in medicine meant that a greater understanding developed regarding the benefits of washing and as cleanliness proved to be linked with better personal health and hygiene so cleansing products began to emerge. Soaps made at home were used to wash clothes and were crudely produced and unfavourable for use on the body. These types of soaps were produced in huge, unattractive slabs from which usable chunks were broken off.

Soon, pharmacists, apothecaries and chemists started to develop products that were functional as well as some with a beauty benefit. Essential oils from different regions of the world were used in creams and soaps not only for their aromas but also for their therapeutic and beautifying properties.

> The company Yardley is famous for its perfumed soaps. As far back as 1620 it received a soap concession from Charles 1 but it took until 1770 for its wares to be available to the wealthier public, with the opening of a shop in London's Bond Street., Yardley soaps are widely available today at a modest price.

And as the pampered royal and wealthy families of the world had greater access to the medical minds of their day, it was proved that to be clean meant greater health and hygiene and therefore, potentially longer life. Even greater emphasis could thus be placed on the attainment of beauty and they set the standards for the rest of the world to follow.

As the Western world progressed scientifically and entered a new age of industry and wealth it became considered developed and civilised. The Eastern cultures, however, clung to their traditions, steeped in mystery and shrouded in mystique and a divide developed which was to last many generations. Now that the boundaries have almost completely opened up and the worlds of beauty more integrated a more homogenised face of beauty is emerging for the future.

Whilst the 19th century saw the beginnings of the beauty industry as trade, travel and knowledge broadened the outlook for health and beauty, the 20th century introduced brands that remain household names of today. Many personalities emerged whose names and the images and ideals they created are still exerting influence in the current highly competitive market.

Innovative, passionate individuals whose close work with the public in pharmacies, perfumeries, salons and movie sets helped them to understand the functional and emotional needs behind the products they were developing for their clients who were becoming increasingly influential and demanding. Companies like Pond's, Rimmel and Guerlain made their debuts in the late 19th century but came into their own in the 20th.

In 1846 Theron Pond a pharmacist from Utica New York introduced Pond's Golden Treasure, a witch hazel based wonder product that went on to be relaunched as Pond's Extract in 1886 before becoming Pond's Cold Cream and Vanishing Cream in 1914. These became the staple of many women's beauty routines. The image of the heavy white porcelain pot with its green lid filled with exotic cream is enough to take me back to my mother's 1950s dressing table where the memory of its distinct odour conjures up for mc all that was beautiful and glamorous at that time. Still available today, albeit at the cheaper end of the market, the pot has become unbreakable and the packaging unremarkable, but the basic ingredients have remained the same. It nonetheless pales into insignificance amongst the higher profile, all singing, all dancing products with their Choose Me packaging, expensive advertising campaigns and price tags to match.

The House of Rimmel was established in 1834 in London. Eugene Rimmel was a French perfumer apprenticed to his father. He experimented with colour and fragrance, developing perfumes, skin care products and makeup for personal hygiene and beauty. From his Regent Street base Rimmel went on to formulate one of the first non-toxic commercial mascaras. In fact, Rimmel is the word for mascara in many languages including Persian, Portuguese, Turkish, Romanian and Spanish.

Pierre Francois Pascal Guerlain studied medicine and chemistry in London and founded Guerlain as a perfume company in 1828. It opened its first beauty salon in Paris in 1939. Over a century later, Guerlain continues to focus on the higher end of cosmetics and perfumery.

Max Factor, Helena Rubinstein, Elizabeth Arden and Charles Revson were all instrumental in taking health and beauty to the next level as health was taken more for granted and beauty aspirations were heightened.

Max Factor was apprenticed with a wigmaker in the late 1800s before being hired by a prominent salon in Berlin. From there he worked with the wigmaker and cosmetician for the Imperial Russian Grand Opera where he developed his skill as a makeup artist. On moving to America in 1904 he opened a store selling makeup, perfume and hair products. By 1914 as well as selling products and giving makeup advice, he also perfected the first makeup for the new motion pictures.

In the first part of the 20th century, Helena Rubinstein and Elizabeth Arden opened exclusive beauty salons in London's fashionable Bond Street producing beauty products and establishing beautifying techniques that went on to be used the world over. However the two doyens of the beauty world maintained a strong personal and professional rivalry that lasted a lifetime.

Charles Revson started Revlon in 1932 specialising in nail enamel from which he made his name. By introducing lipsticks that matched the enamels he assured himself a place in beauty history before adding to his range of cosmetics and perfumes - most notably Charlie - an affordable scent which changed the face of perfumery.

These people did not invent any new products but adapted and developed what was already available. What they did do was change the perception of beauty by channelling their passion into the new art and practice of advertising their products. Before legislation was enforced, many of the claims they made were at best unfounded and at worst untrue, but were none the less instrumental in creating a desire for as well as meeting the need for beauty that has taken these companies into the new millennium.

Haute couture got in on the act, with key players using their names to launch high-end beauty products and fragrances. People such as Coco Chanel, Christian Dior and Yves Saint Laurent helped create a hype that fuelled the desire and developed a yearning for beauty that grew to obsessive heights.

Coco Chanel opened her own millinery shop in 1910 and went on to change women's fashion for all time. Her signature perfume Chanel Number 5 made its debut in 1921, the same year in which she also made for herself the first stick of the blood red lip colour that was to become her cosmetic trademark.

Christian Dior launched his glamorous and controversial New Look in 1947, which was aspired to by every woman despite the difficult economic times. Perfumes furthered his reputation for luxury, which were followed with cosmetics and skin care.

In 1955 Yves Saint Laurent worked as a young designer at Christian Dior taking over after Dior's death two years later. In 1962 he opened his own couture house to enormous acclaim and went on to introduce perfumes, skin care and makeup.

Further development saw companies and products merge to gain greater control over the market, whilst still retaining the names and reflecting the images of their founders. Creators of beauty became celebrities and pioneers as the likes of Estée Lauder, Mary Quant and Anita Roddick joined their ranks.

> Estée Lauder started her company in 1946 with four products declaring that 'every woman can be beautiful'. Selling her products in department stores, Estée Lauder soon established a loyal following, with many of her skin care, makeup and perfumes enjoying cult status. She increased her notoriety with the launch of the popular men's Aramis range. Estée Lauder's products remain a firm favourite today commanding prestigious floor space in department stores worldwide.
>
> In the 1960s Mary Quant launched the mini skirt as part of the Swinging Sixties, helping to establish London as the centre of creative fashion. 1966 saw the introduction of Mary Quant cosmetics designed for young women as a natural compliment to her fashion line.
>
> Anita Roddick opened the first Body Shop store in Brighton in 1976 and went on to become a global manufacturer and retailer of naturally inspired and ethically produced beauty and cosmetic products.

Products moved from being purely functional to providing beauty benefits in an industry whose massive growth and development was instrumental in not only meeting the growing need in people for beautification but also in precipitating trends by developing strong links with fashion.

A phenomenon was created which took on a life of its own. It was to become one of the richest and fastest growing global industries, a success which shows no signs of letting up. What was once seen as an industry for 'outsiders' has become acceptable at all levels. Products that were once viewed with scepticism have become necessary components of daily grooming. The face paints and pastes of the past have emerged as the latest 'must have' accessories along with handbags, shoes and jewellery. Perfumes no longer disguise unpleasant aromas; instead they take men as well as women everywhere from work place to leisure pursuits on fragrant mood enhancing, image making journeys through the realms of beauty.

Not only do we now have better health but also the potential for greater beauty and as health and hygiene have added credibility to grooming , celebrity endorsement has ensured that the beautification of the body is acceptable at all levels of society.

Technology has brought with it many innovations, and the results can be seen in improved lifestyles and raised personal expectations and aspirations. As trade, travel and education have improved so too has choice, so there is no longer any need to search for beauty. It finds us.

It cannot be denied that for better or for worse, in good times and in bad, for richer and poorer, howsoever we perceive it, beauty matters.

Beauty is a combination of qualities that the senses take pleasure from and the mind exalts - but if beauty is all in the brain can it be found in a tub or a tube?

The legislation associated with recent years has gone a long way towards ensuring that the products on sale today live up to their claims. It is a fact that the listed ingredients of any product have all been scientifically proven to be of value, that the sell by and use by dates ascertain their longevity and we may be safe in the knowledge that they have been thoroughly tried and tested before reaching the point of sale. Celebrity endorsements through innovative advertising adds to the credibility of the products we buy and word of mouth is enhanced by the increasing use of a social media that is a world away from that which launched the beauty industry of the past.

But is it the truth, the whole truth and nothing but the truth?

Whilst science and technology are attempting to take care of our physical beauty needs with the development of pioneering products, our psychological desires are seduced by groundbreaking methods of communication through social media networking.

The lotions and potions of the past have been tweaked and twittered to such an extent that reality recedes as more and more tubs and tubes not only overflow our bathroom cabinets, but gather dust on bedroom dressing tables. No sooner do we finish one product than we are on to the next.

Mesmerising images are brought to mind by the mere squeeze of a tube whilst promises of the elixir within sets the senses alight. No amount of disappointment dampens our enthusiasm as we move on to the next product taking in our stride the hype whilst trying to decipher the jargon.

We yoyo between resurfacing the skin with AHAs, fighting free radical attack with antioxidants, improving skin clarity with Retinol, rejuvenating with pentapeptides, hydrating and restoring with hyaluronic acid and fortifying with EFAs with a confidence that belies our intelligence. Each new innovation taking us deeper into the realms of beauty as never before, often without any understanding of the physiological needs of our skins as we feed the psychological with the feel good factor that accompanies each new product purchase and its associated beauty ideal.

Glossary of Terms

- **AHAs** – Alpha Hydroxy Acids also referred to as fruit acids, derived from sugar cane in the form of glycolic acid, from citrus fruits as citric acid and from milk as lactic acid. Natural exfoliators that break down the substance binding the skin cells together.
- **Free Radicals** – the toxic by product of energy production responsible for ageing. Pollution, cigarette smoke and ultra violet rays are examples of free radicals.

- **Antioxidants** – substances capable of guarding the skin against free radical attack eg vitamins A, C and E.

- **Pentapeptides** – a peptide is a particle of protein and pentapeptides refers to chains of peptides. Protein is essential for the repair and renewal of skin cells.

- **Retinol** – a pure form of vitamin A which as well as being an antioxidant, stimulates cell renewal helping to improve texture and tone.

- **Hyaluronic acid** – also known as glycosaminoglycan and capable of absorbing water like a sponge acting as an humectant helping to keep skin hydrated and youthful.

- **EFAs** – Essential Fatty Acids in the form of Omegas 3 and 6 which combat inflammation as well as strengthen the skin cells.

Even when you strip away the celebrity hype, unravel the mysteries surrounding the over use of jargon and remove the Choose Me packaging there is beauty to be found in the tubs and tubes on sale today.

However, whether or not the beauty we are buying is the right one for us and can deliver the one our hearts and minds desire comes down to perception. Through perception there is the opportunity for a sensorial journey to explore beauty via physical, psychological and spiritual means and establish what lies behind its various dimensions to discover its ultimate and intimate truth.

Let the journey begin.

Perception

CHAPTER TWO

Sight

If the sight of the blue skies fills you with joy,
if a blade of grass springing up in the fields has
power to move you, if the simple things of
nature have a message that you understand,
rejoice, for your soul is alive.

Eleonora Duse

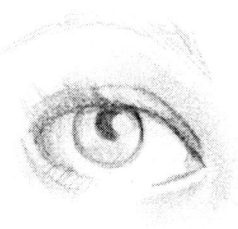 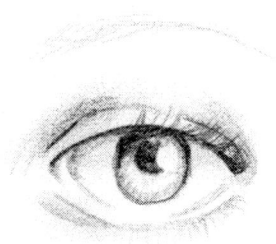

The Science of Sight

The eyes' sensory function takes up a large part of the brain, beginning within the occipital lobe where information is received from the eyes via the optic cranial nerves in the form of patterns of light, which are then drawn up into a kind of map. This information is subsequently transported to various different parts of the brain to be analysed into recognisable colours, objects, people and places. This function facilitates the recognition of physical beauty, has a close association with first impressions and as such is the sensory function that has the most impact and is heavily relied upon in order to evaluate outer beauty.

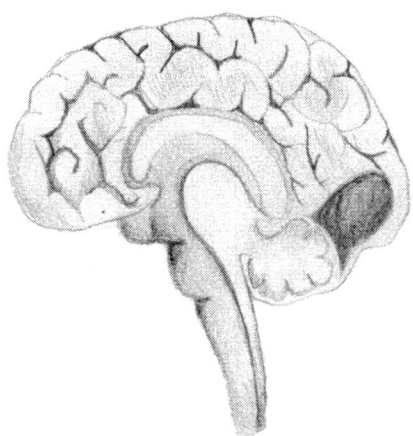

SENSE OF SIGHT

The Art of Sight

Clairvoyance (clear vision) is one of the extra sensory functions enabling a person to gain information about an object, person or place by means other than the physical and is often referred to as second sight.

Energy from the past or future is believed to manifest itself in such a way as to be seen by the mind's eye as an unexplained vision. This visual energy may appear in the form of dream, a *déjà vu*, as part of a meditative practice or as a random vision and is often linked to some kind of foresight or warning. Clairvoyance is one of the more accepted of the extra sensory functions although there still exists much cynicism surrounding its reliability and criticism of its use and in some circumstances, abuse. Clairvoyance provides the opportunity to view the beauty that lies beyond that which the eyes alone can see.

The eyes are said to be the most important feature of the face and are believed to reflect the soul.

They offer an insight into the rest of the body not only as a window into the soul but also as a reflection of the body as a whole. Iridology refers to the study of the iris of the eye in order to diagnose disease within the body. The body systems and individual organs are mapped out in a chart of the iris which like a clock face may be divided into 12 segments, with each segment relating to specific area of the body. Changes in the pattern and colour within each section relates directly to the associated body part with iridologists able to make an interpretation and from that form a diagnosis.

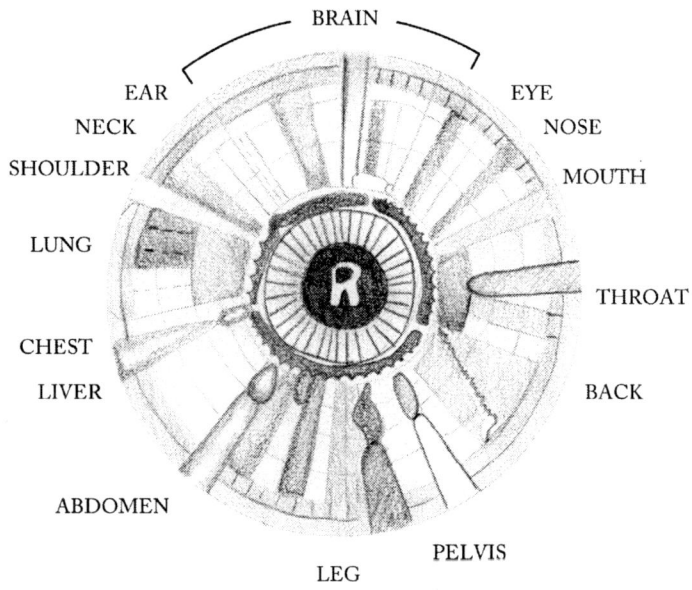

Eye Facts - The Physical Eye

The eyes are contained within the sockets created by the bones of the skull. Each eye is shaped like a small ball and contains the cornea, iris, pupil and retina. The cornea is responsible for receiving light, which is then regulated by the iris as the pupil alters its size to accommodate the incoming rays. The light sensitive cells contained in the retina convert the light rays into electrical impulses before being sent to the brain via the optic nerves. The circular *orbicularis occuli* muscles surround each eye and contribute to the formation of crow's feet - the fine lines and wrinkles that appear as the muscle slackens with age, use and abuse - whilst the *corrugator supercilli* muscles are responsible for drawing together the eyebrows to form a vertical frown of concentration that will in time become an ingrained stress line. These muscles help to form some of the facial expressions vital to our non-verbal methods of communication.

Each eye contains a tear duct and gland known as the lacrimal gland that produces a cleansing fluid and is activated not only as a means to clear the eye of unwanted substances and keep it well hydrated but also as an expression of extreme emotion. Further protection is offered to the eyes by the hair of the eyelashes and eyebrows. Eye colour develops during early childhood as the colour pigment melanin is produced that determines the eye colour. Babies are mostly born with unpigmented eyes.

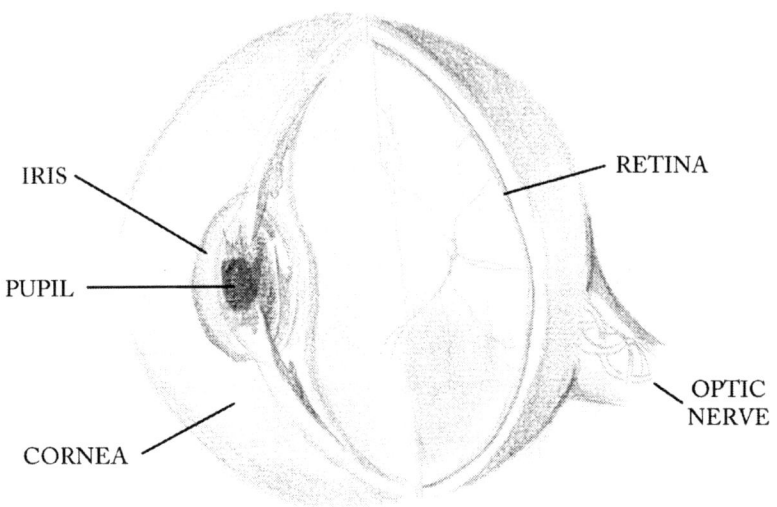

IRIS

PUPIL

CORNEA

RETINA

OPTIC
NERVE

Eye Facts - The Emotional Eye

The eyes bare a strong link with a person's emotions and as such are capable of demonstrating extreme levels of sentiment through the production of tears. The lacrimal glands of the eyes are able to produce three different types of tear:

- **Basal** tears that are being constantly produced to keep the eyes hydrated and remain within the eyes

- **Reflex** tears that are produced in response to irritation helping to flush out foreign particles

- **Psychic** tears that are produced as part of an exclusive human function associated with emotional crying

Different parts of the brain initiate the production of the tear types with the ability to produce psychic tears remaining inactive until some time after birth. This process develops further with emotional stimulation and memory and remains active throughout life. However, the act of crying psychic tears holds social prejudices and may on the one hand be seen as a useful means of emotional release whilst being a sign of emotional weakness on the other.

Eye Facts – The Spiritual Eye

In addition to the physical and emotional eyes there also exists the concept of a third eye that has a spiritual connection. The third eye forms part of the chakra system, is also known as the brow chakra and has strong associations with the colour indigo. Situated in the space between the eyebrows it is believed to be capable of intuitive vision. It is said that this eye helps to forge the visible links with spirituality examples of which include the 'seeing' of colours or images that may accompany the art of clairvoyance.

The principles surrounding the spiritual third eye come in the main from the Eastern beliefs associated with Chinese Traditional Medicine and Ayurveda, belief systems which focus on the idea of an energy system that exists to link the body with all that surrounds it and vice versa. Energy in the form of light enters and exits the body via the seven main chakras.

> From the Sanskrit word meaning vortexes of energy chakras are often referred to as being wheels of light.

Light is supplied by the energy of the sun of which all life is dependent upon and the seven colours of the rainbow are contained within its rays. The energy associated with each colour resonates with a different wavelength and at varying frequencies and is able to enter and exit the body via one of the seven chakras. The seven colours of the rainbow are linked with the seven main chakras as follows:

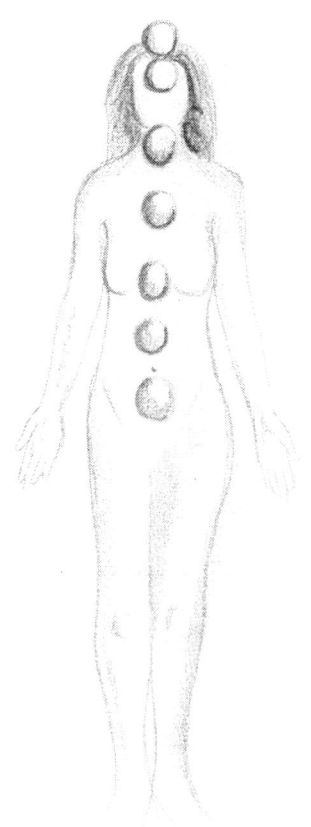

The crown chakra – violet

The brow or third eye chakra – indigo

The throat chakra - blue

The heart chakra - green

The solar plexus chakra - yellow

The sacral chakra – orange

The base chakra – red

The energy that radiates from each chakra is believed to have a spiritual effect on the corresponding parts of the body as well as be affected by the physiology and psychology of the area it services, that is, how a part of the body feels and how we feel about it.

Therefore, each chakra has a link to the physical and the emotional as well the spiritual. This holistic viewpoint subscribes to the concept that the part can never be well unless the whole is well and forms the basis of many holistic beauty treatments.

Colour

Colour is light with different wavelengths and frequencies.

The spectrum of visible colours is contained in the white light from the sun. The energy associated with each colour has the potential to provide a physical, emotional and spiritual effect on the body.

- Violet: the highest colour in the visible spectrum with the lowest wavelength but the highest frequency. Violet is classified as a cool colour with a calming effect on the body and mind being associated with a sense of bliss, understanding and enlightenment encouraging and supporting cosmic awareness, self realisation and spirituality. Violet is associated with the crown chakra

- Indigo: the next colour in the spectrum. It is also classified as being a cool colour and has a sedative effect, which supports and strengthens our dreams encouraging the development of intuition and inner vision cultivating our imagination and the projection of will by mental power. Indigo is associated with the brow or third eye chakra

- Blue: following indigo in the spectrum, blue is a cool colour with a relaxing effect initiating the power of self expression by connecting with knowledge of our past, present and future and using our inner voice to communicate and inspire. Blue is associated with the throat chakra

- Green: in the middle of the spectrum and as such may be classified as both a cool and a warm colour. Green is associated with balance and harmony in all things providing the natural links between science and art through unconditional love, devotion, passion and compassion. Green is associated with the heart chakra

- Yellow: following green in the spectrum, yellow is a warm colour providing a stimulating effect through which shines the radiance of identity, power and strength forming an integration of feelings and experiences. Yellow is associated with the solar plexus chakra

- Orange: next in the colour spectrum and as another warm colour it has energising properties that fuel fertility, creativity, productivity through spontaneous cleansing, purification and release. Orange is associated with the sacral chakra.

- Red: the lowest colour in the spectrum with the highest wavelength and lowest frequency. A warm colour with exciting and powerful properties that encourage mental and physical stability and control through sexuality, passion and survival. Red is associated with the base chakra.

> Historically rouge and red lip tints are probably amongst the most widely used cosmetics of all time due to the wavelengths and frequencies associated with the colour red which gives it the ability to stimulate the greatest subconscious response.

Advances in the feel good factor associated with traditional beauty treatments have initiated the acceptance of further holistic therapies in recent years. For some this is seen as being an extension of the beauty industry whilst for others it forms a separate branch of business with a completely different mindset. Beauty therapy is often viewed as being the superficial branch associated with outer beauty whist holistic therapy is classified as operating at a deeper level focusing on inner beauty.

However, if we look good on a superficial level we more often than not feel good at a deeper level If we feel good at a deep level we more often than not look better at a superficial level.

It may be suggested that you cannot have one without the other and that is exactly what the traditions of Chinese Medicine and the Ayurvedic paradigm are all about, ie balance.

The third eye chakra and its associations with the colour indigo has the ability to develop a greater level of inner vision and so the potential to have a more balanced view of beauty as a whole.

The ability to make use of the emotional and spiritual eyes in addition to the physical eyes facilitates the recognition of psychological and spiritual beauty, which has subtler and less quantifiable associations with first impressions and as such are sensory functions that are often unused and misunderstood and so ignored yet may be used to evaluate inner beauty.

Eye Beauty

The iris should fill a large space in the eye and be of a distinct colour. The whites of the eyes should be clear and bright and the pupils should shine and twinkle.

Eyes should be fringed with long lashes and framed by well-defined brows.

According to the rules of symmetry, the ideal female eyes lie in the middle third of the face in line with the top of the ears. There should be an eye width space between each eye with the eyebrow placed slightly above the upper orbital rim with a prominent arch located at the level of the outer rim of the pupil. The upper lid should have its highest point a third of the width of the eye away from the inner corner and the lower lid should have its lowest point a third of the width of an eye away from the outer corner. The upper lid should slightly cover the top of the iris whilst the lower lid allows the lower portion of the iris to be visible.

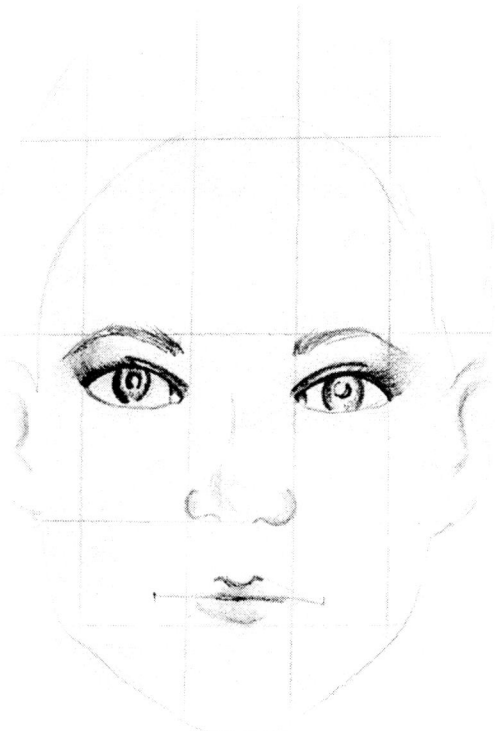

THE PERFECT EYE

The start of the eyebrows may be measured from a vertical line taken from the corner of the nose to meet the inner corner of the eye and beyond with the end of the brow appearing as a diagonal line is taken from the corner of the nose to meet the outer corner of the eye and beyond.

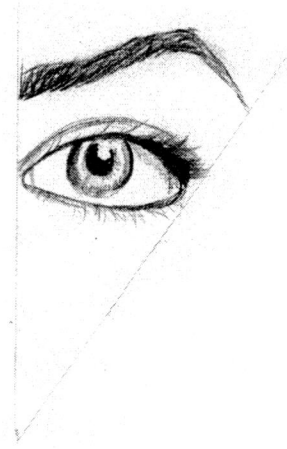

THE PERFECT EYEBROW

The ideal male eyes will be similarly placed with the eyebrows lying fairly flat at the upper orbital rim.

Whilst the eyes and eyebrows contribute to physical symmetry and thus outer beauty they are also thought to be associated with the balance of the yin and yang energy and thus inner beauty.

Yin and yang refer to the female and male energies and attributes with the left eye having an association with the female yin energy and the right eye with the male yang energy.

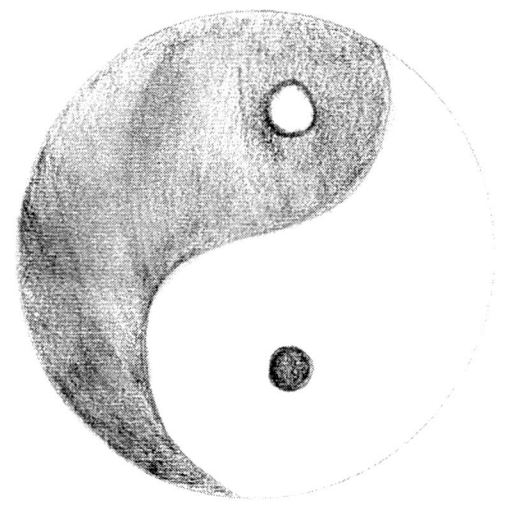

YIN AND YANG

Qualities of Yin	Qualities of Yang
Feminine	*Masculine*
Moon	*Sun*
Dark	*Light*
Shade	*Bright*
Sunset	*Sunrise*
Earth	*Heaven*
Rest	*Activity*
Water	*Fire*
Cold	*Heat*
Front of body	*Back of body*
Internal body	*External body*
Structure	*Function*
Deficiency	*Excess*
Hypo activity	*Hyperactivity*

Yin and yang form a fundamental part of Chinese Traditional Medicine. They are opposite and interdependent – there is not one without the other.

Close and/or deep-set eyes with brows that slant towards the bridge of the nose are believed to reflect greater yang tendencies in a person whilst eyes that are further spaced and protruding with brows that slant away from the nose demonstrate greater yin tendencies. Inner beauty is reflected in a balance between the yin and yang energies in much the same way, as outer beauty is dependent on the idea of perfect physical symmetry.

Eye Power

The eyes form an integral part of the beauty picture. Not only do they see beauty, they also reflect it. As such the eyes become both the beholder and the holder of beauty, providing a powerful means of communication.

The mind relies on the eyes to communicate a vision for it to interpret and produce a suitable response. This facility changes throughout the cycles of life:

- A small child looks at the world with an open mind and reacts to the differences it sees without prejudice or judgment. Beauty has an innocence and may be found in all they see
- Puberty brings with it the vision of the ideal mate firmly lodged in the mind's eye, as hormones become

responsible for initiating the need to seek the most suitable partner with whom to procreate. Beauty becomes selective, seductive and as a result, stressful

- Menopause and the male equivalent andropause results in a drop in hormone levels with the resulting mindset often at odds with the reality as changes in the body happen before the mind is willing to accept them. Beauty loses its energy but maintains its momentum becoming more associated with stress and less about selection and seduction

The eyes act as both attractors and detractors. Beautiful eyes are able to detract attention away from less attractive areas of the face. The health of the body and the sharpness of the mind may be communicated through the eyes both of which contain strong elements of beauty which may be used as sign posts for selection, indications of attraction and a means of seduction.

The eyes have a long association with makeup to enhance their beauty powers.

> Colour is artfully used to create and/or recreate the beauty of the eyes with the use of eye shadow. Colours may be chosen intuitively as a reflection of inner beauty and/or with the intention of enhancing outer beauty.

The Language of the Eyes

The eyes say it all without words.

Eyes light up with pleasure, widen with surprise, crease with laughter, screw up with pain, water with emotion, soften with love, flash with anger, twinkle with mystery. It is little wonder that they are referred to as windows to the soul and why many people feel the need to hide behind a long fringe or a pair of oversized sunglasses. As part of the 'fight or flight' syndrome pupils dilate when a person is taken out of their comfort zone and faced with something unexpected eg when we come face to face with someone we find attractive our pupils will dilate.

The ability to maintain good eye contact shows interest, politeness and sincerity, demonstrating the self-confidence that accompanies a positive outlook. Conversely a lack of eye contact not only communicates lack of interest, rudeness and insincerity but also is also a symptom of poor self-esteem and a reflection of low levels of self-confidence. However, in some cultures too much eye contact is seen as brazen whilst a lack of constant eye contact demonstrates respect and a more demure demeanour.

Eyebrows contribute to human methods of non-verbal communication with the ability to express emotions and sentiments. Eyebrows that rise and fall express feelings associated with happiness whilst when held low and close to the eyes feelings of discontent are demonstrated. Eyebrows lift with surprise, draw together with concern and are even able to rise singularly when feelings of imbalance and confusion set in. Aggression is often communicated when eyebrows have been pierced which may or may not be reflected in behaviour.

The eyes and eyebrows have the ability to speak the unspoken bypassing the brain rather like a reflex action and in this way offer a glimpse of truth before the mind has time to think things through. The eyes retain a childlike reaction to beauty that the mind lacks when judgment takes over.

> Eyes show beauty when they reflect thoughts that are beautiful. Beauty, charm and power are lost when jealousy, envy, cunning and suspicion are depicted in the eyes.

Eye Care

The eyes, eyebrows and surrounding skin require special care to maintain their function and beauty.

Water intake contributes to the fluid levels of the eyes and the surrounding skin, which needs to remain well hydrated at all times for comfort and protection.

> **Waterworks:** All cells are made up of approximately 70% water, which gets used up as the cells perform their various functions and needs to be regularly replenished if cells are to perform to their optimum.

Rest is necessary for the eyes to stay clear. Even during waking hours it is still necessary to rest the eyes from time to time. Closing them for a moment is soothing and calming, letting them wander at distance eases them whilst allowing them to glaze over in a daydream is both physically and mentally relaxing.

> In yoga, *drishtis* or gazes are used to direct the eyes whilst practising a posture or *asana*. This has a calming and relaxing effect by developing greater focus resulting in increased concentration and mind control.

Regular eye tests ensure vision is corrected as necessary and eyestrain is avoided. Opticians and iridologists are able to detect the warning signs of more serious diseases through the analysis of the eyes that affect the whole body providing greater potential for cure.

Beauty Vision:

- Contact lenses can change eye colour as well as correct sight
- Glasses wearers can choose frames that compliment eye and face shape as well as enhancing their colouring
- Sunglasses shield the eyes creating an ideal sunscreen

Eye makeup needs to be applied and removed with care. The skin surrounding the eyes is finer than that of the rest of the face and body and reacts badly to being dragged, pulled or prodded.

> **Makeup Facts:** Eye makeup beyond its use by date, shared amongst friends or applied with implements or fingers that are unclean are common causes of eye infections, irritations and allergies.

Mascara, false lashes, lash extensions, tints and perms should be used with caution to prevent loss of lashes and irritation to the eyes. Sensitivity tests need to be carried out prior to the use of chemicals to avoid allergic reactions that may be potentially damaging to the eyes.

> **Sensitivity Tests:** These should be carried out prior to any chemical being used on the eyes eg tint, glue, perm solution. A small amount of the product is placed onto the cleansed skin of a sensitive part of the body (often behind the ear) and left to react. An adverse reaction will result in inflammation and irritation to the surrounding skin, which may or may not affect the rest of the body. Further application of the product to the eye area must in this case be avoided with treatment only taking place if there was no reaction after testing.

Cleanliness and hygiene are vital for the well being of the eyes and surrounding skin. Eyebaths rinse away irritation, eye makeup removers dissolve makeup and clean implements prevent infection.

> **Eye Care:** Dry cotton wool should be avoided when removing makeup from the eye area as the tiny fibres can enter the eye and/or cause damage to the surrounding skin. Always use damp cotton wool pads and cotton buds.
>
> Cleanse eyes in a circular motion working in over the eyelashes of closed eyes and out over the brow area. Any particles of eye makeup that enter the eyes are easily flushed out via the inner corner avoiding undue irritation.

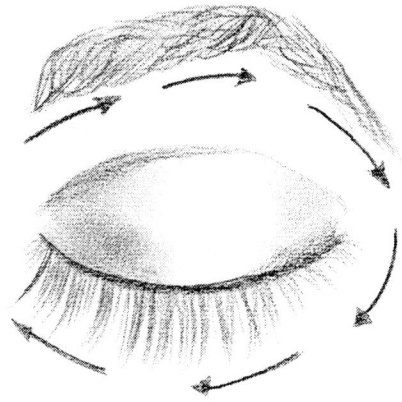

CLEANSING OF THE EYES

To combat the signs of aging specific eye gels and creams are recommended to nourish the surrounding skin, soothe away dark circles, eliminate puffiness as well as soften the appearance of lines and wrinkles. Exposure to UV light should be minimal and smoking should be avoided completely as both are the major contributors to premature ageing of the eyes and surrounding skin.

Anti Ageing Eye

Face or body moisturisers are not suitable for the eye area and should be avoided in place of specific eye gels and creams.

Eye gels are cooling and soothing and generally used to treat young eyes as prevention to ageing.

Eye creams provide more nourishment and are suited to eyes that are beginning to show the signs of ageing.

> Both gels and creams should be applied following some basic guidelines:
>
> - Men can benefit from eye gels or creams as much as women
> - Apply in the morning alone or under eye makeup
> - Apply in the evening after washing or removal of eye makeup
> - Use ring fingers to apply for gentle pressure
> - Apply around the eye in a circular motion avoiding the upper eyelid and lower eye lip
> - Avoid using too much product as this can block pores and irritate the eyes
> - Place any excess cream on and around the lips as the skin in this area will benefit greatly from the application of such a product

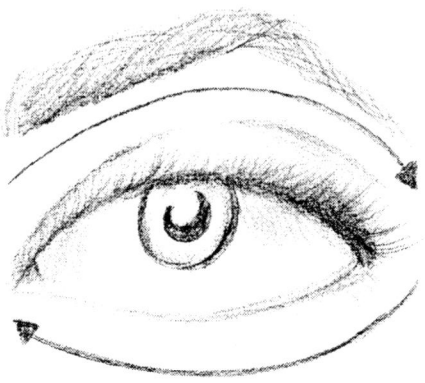

APPLICATION OF EYE GEL/CREAM

Careful eyebrow shaping can change the appearance of face shape helping to create the illusion of the ideal oval shaped face.

Eyebrow Shapes

- Flat eyebrows shorten a long face shape
- High arched eyebrows lengthen a round face shape
- Thick defined eyebrows balance a heavy jaw or square face shape
- Rounded eyebrows compliment a heart face shape. A low arch shortens a long shape and a high arch lengthens a short shape
- Curved eyebrows even out the harsh lines of a diamond face shape creating a softer effect

Great care should be taken when removing hairs from the eyebrows to achieve the ideal shape. Plucking, waxing and threading are all popular methods of hair removal that require careful consideration prior to and post use. It is worth bearing in mind that skin sensitivity levels rise during menstruation and when the body is stressed or unwell so such treatments are best avoided during these times.

Eyebrow Care

Hair removal is an aggressive treatment on the skin, which should be carried out with care and attention to detail to avoid discomfort and trauma.

Plucking:

- Tweezers should be clean and in good working order
- Tweezers for removing single hairs may be flat ended, pointed or slanted
- Automatic tweezers may be used to remove multiple hairs
- The eyebrows and surrounding skin should be clean and dry and a warm compress applied to open pores
- Always tweeze hairs from their base and in the direction of growth holding the surrounding skin taut to avoid bruising and to minimise stimulation to the underlying blood supply
- Apply a cooling lotion or toner post tweezing to close pores and calm the skin.

Waxing and threading are best left to the experts as painful and unattractive mistakes are common, and both methods require skill and artistic experience in their execution.

Special Care

The eyes, eyebrows and surrounding skin take immense comfort and gain great benefit from special care. Time taken caring for the eyes will add to and enhance the beauty of a person as that care is reflected in the eyes.

Eye masks offer special care to the eyes and surrounding area and are available in many varied forms including:

Prescriptive eye masks that form part of a salon treatment targeting specific problems

Shop bought premixed masks that can be applied at home. Best applied when relaxing.

Home-made masks that offer a natural and inexpensive alternative to the above. Soak cotton wool pads in an infusion of:

- Weak black tea – used to stimulate and revive.

- Rose water – used to soothe and calm.

- Lettuce and cucumber juice – used to tighten and tone

Textured eye masks worn to block out the light can add to the special care of the eyes aiding specific problems as well as promoting peaceful sleep and calming relaxation:

- Cashmere eye masks offer a soft and gentle covering to eyes reducing stress and strain

- Perfumed eye cushions containing dried lavender, rose petals etc. add a gentle and soothing pressure to the eyes, helping to prevent dark circles

- Cooling masks that have been refrigerated prior to use tighten, refine and help to reduce puffiness

The emotional eye benefits from being permitted to express core feelings, especially those associated with anger, frustration and grief through the production of psychic tears. The physical act of crying enables these feelings to be aired, accepted and released. Psychic tears have the action of flushing out such feelings and help you to regain a greater sense of emotional balance.

Psychic Tears: Giving in to the act of crying can help to alleviate the pain associated with emotional baggage that can weigh heavily within the mind, often manifesting itself in heavy physical symptoms. Relaxation makes it possible for the mind and body to let go with crying often a direct result. Whilst this may be viewed in a negative light, it can be extremely positive as the flushed out emotions are replaced with a sense of lightness that is both healing and restorative.

Spiritual Care

The spiritual, third eye also benefits from special care helping to keep the channels of energy free flowing enhancing levels of inner beauty with the potential to create greater levels of overall balance and harmony.

The simple practice of breath work, meditation and visualisations all contribute to the inner well being of the third eye chakra and may be used as a powerful tool to re energise, rejuvenate and regenerate.

Breath work: breathe deeply in through the nose and out through the mouth for three breaths.

> Meditation: with each inward and outward breath focus the mind on drawing the air in and out of the third eye situated between the eyebrows.
>
> Visualisation: create a visual image of brightness entering the third eye with the inward breath allowing any dull or murky energy to exit with the outward breath.

Beauty will reflect and be reflected in the physical, emotional and spiritual care the eyes enjoy throughout a person's lifetime.

Visual Beauty

Beauty is intrinsically linked with image and whilst the theory of beauty remains unchanged the visual face of beauty is ever changing.

Throughout time ideal images of feminine and masculine beauty have been held up to the masses for all to see and emulate regardless of suitability, practicality and sensibility.

Beauty becomes a vision that is looked at with the eyes yet seen with the mind.

Images and Reflections

As the image of perfect beauty is mostly associated with fertility it is not surprising that for many, beauty is synonymous with youth. The older we get, the younger we are encouraged to appear and as our life expectancy has increased so has the desire to not only once again reinvent beauty for a new generation, but to apply greater and greater pressure on achieving and maintaining its youthful image. As we continue to create a false reality by chasing this impossible dream are we in danger of losing our identity?

One explanation for our preoccupation with youth may be found in the advancing technology and changing lifestyles associated with the early 20th century. As candlelight gave way to electric light faces and bodies were highlighted as never before.

This was further compounded by the invention of moving pictures and the subsequent presentation of movie stars who were picked as much for their physical beauty as for their talent. The ordinary person was able to see their idols on the big screen. This inevitably led to comparison and the human desire to emulate became ever stronger.

Fan magazines, beauty columns and product advertisements cultivated this desire in the ordinary person to emulate what they saw. The average person was not only seeing more images of the stars they wanted to be like, they were also seeing more reflections of themselves with the mass production of mirrors and the invention of cameras.

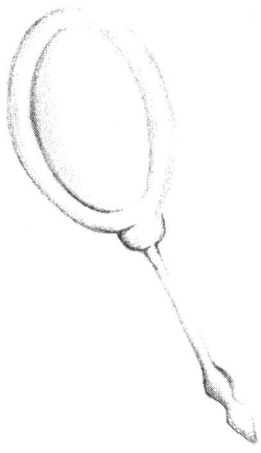

MIRROR

Once a luxury of the wealthy, mirrors were now everywhere. They were even used to advertise a whole host of products as businesses gave away pocket mirrors with their logo or slogan on the back in an attempt to promote their wares in an innovative way.

The invention and subsequent boom in the use of cameras meant that not only were real life images of the stars on view as picture magazines increased in circulation and popularity, but ordinary people were able to take snapshots of themselves and their loved ones.

It is hard for us to imagine the impact this had. The resulting emotional predicament as people found their image to be inevitably wanting and increasingly waning was to fuel the beauty industry and it is at this time that we see massive advancements in the development and marketing of cosmetics.

This had an effect on all corners of society.

The wealthy upper classes could seek professional help. Beauty salons opened, the up and coming middle classes began to buy into this world with affordable mail order products and mass production brought products into the budgets of poorer people. Whilst the years of the first and second world wars hindered this progress they by no means halted it. The traditional roles and attitudes of women changed and the post war beauty boom that followed was to last to the present day.

As a direct result of the war, advancements in surgery were made to assist in the reconstruction of and recovery from horrific wounds. The ensuing technology was used, and some might say abused, in the quest to turn back time; the first facelifts were performed in the early 20th century.

Since then we haven't looked back as greater chemical research and medical experience has broadened knowledge and skill and more and more products and procedures are widely available. Developments in technology initiated the use of computerised enhancement to produce the beauty images that adorn the endless pages of today's popular magazines, which have a closer association with science fiction than real life.

Bogus Beauty

As a direct result of the advances made in science and technology, post pubescent physical perfection is held up as the perfect model of beauty in much the same way as it is viewed as being the prerequisite for perfect health.

As the never ending and ever increasing fashion for fake sees hair, nails and lashes extending beyond that which is humanly possible, skin changing colour at the flick of a switch and features being changed beyond all recognition, a mutant form of beauty is fast emerging as faces and bodies are fashioned with a scalpel, augmented with silicone, filled with Botox and implanted with harvested fat. This form of beauty isn't merely about moving the hands of time it is more about developing an exaggerated caricature and is becoming increasingly accessible, affordable and acceptable.

Or is it?

Could this bogus beauty be fast approaching its sell by date or are we just extending the time in which it is used? And if so what will beauty turn into?

Real Radiance versus Fake Fad

How is it that we can look at an old tree and marvel at the radiance of its beauty and yet not see that same level of beauty in an ageing human being?

How is it that the ancient tree conjures up for us a romantic image of a life rich in experience containing a wealth of knowledge within its withered branches when the wrinkles of a maturing woman are not viewed with the same mind's eye?

We stare at the old tree in wonderment marvelling at its age and beauty yet at the same time we shrink away from a woman of lesser years with feelings of distaste. Whilst our tree seems to weather the storms of time with grace and beauty, the beauty of the human race is seen to be ravaged by those very same storms.

> Wrinkles are merely wisdom in disguise.

Beauty has long been linked with perfection and the origins of this ideal may be found in the development and subsequent use of the adjective beautiful which in its classical Greek form was associated with *being of one's hour*. This makes perfect sense if we subscribe to the school of thought that believes that beauty equates to the survival of the species. Being of one's hour could be interpreted as being fully formed, ripe and fertile: at the peak of our ability to attract, seduce and reproduce.

To this end the most beautiful are the winners. This theory pays tribute to the outer beauty associated with the physical that often results in spontaneity, passion and mindless procreation as nature takes over in its purist and most primitive form. However, being of one's hour has a limited time scale in the average person's lifespan especially as we can now expect to live many years beyond our fertility use by date and unfortunately for us we are all too often deemed to be less than beautiful and certainly no longer of our hour long before that cut off date arrives.

The most popular solution to this age-old problem has always been to fake it– to create the illusion that we are still of our hour even when the ability to reproduce has been taken away from us.

The fashion for fake is not a new fad. Wheresoever an image has failed to live up to real or perceived perfection, attempts have been made to realise it. As a result mistakes have inevitably occurred resulting in mutilation, gross deformity and even death. And when perfection is achieved, it is predictably short lived and not without massive risks. Where is the beauty in that?

Neck rings are popular even today within in some tribes of the world. Added gradually, these have the effect of lengthening the neck to inhuman proportions. The more rings, the longer the neck appears. The bearer of the unnaturally lengthened neck has decreasing levels of mobility and a greater expectation of associated health risks.

Foot binding made popular by the Chinese stunted the natural growth of females' feet so that bones were unable to grow normally. Beautiful small feet were the primary aim but the attainment of this level of beauty brought with it constant pain and eventual inability to walk. Girls grew into women with feet that could no longer bear their weight or maintain the body's balance.

Breast enhancement was made popular in the 20th century. Poor surgery has resulted in hideous and unnecessary scars, over-enhancement has put additional and needless strain on the body and inserted products have interfered with the body's natural harmony and caused avoidable reactions that have affected the health of the whole body.

The current trend for injectable fillers has seen facial features changed beyond recognition with trout pouts becoming commonplace.

However bad the consequences are of faking it people are increasingly willing to give it a go and as long as there are products and procedures available there will be people wanting them.

No sooner is one product or procedure made available there comes another that claims to offer bigger, better and quicker or smoother, clearer and faster and even higher, tighter and for longer. A tsunami of products and procedures threaten to overwhelm natural beauty. Will the landscape of beauty be changed forever or is there a reality check on the horizon? Is it enough to create the illusion of beauty by using a brush and palette or is it wholly dependent on the creation of a sham of plastic parts?

Amongst many there is the opinion that when makeup is artfully applied, beauty does not fade but is increased.

Evidence of makeup use has been found in Egypt dating back long before the birth of Christ, and thereafter all over the world archaeologists unearth many relics and artefacts pertaining to the application of products and procedures.

The red and yellow of ochre, powdered saffron, dried red wine and berry juice, the grey/black of charcoal and ash and the white of chalk and lead have all been used in the popular colour palettes of ancient times. Plant dyes darkened eyebrows whilst vinegar and beer have lightened hair. Crude implements to mix and apply makeup were made out of plants, wood and metal.

Historians have been able to add to the strength and validity of this evidence with facts of their own. However, the history of the use of makeup is shrouded in controversy, contradiction and change.

> The Roman playwright Plautus is said to have declared that a woman without paint is like food without salt.
>
> Queen Victoria once stated that makeup was improper, vulgar and acceptable only for actors.
>
> Adolph Hitler is reported to have said that makeup was for clowns and not women of the master race.

Throughout the years makeup has contributed to both the creation and reflection of beauty. It is a shroud behind which a person can hide their real selves.

It is a tool with which the blank canvas can reflect the many and varied faces of both the internal and external beauty of an individual at each stage of their life cycle.

For me makeup serves to meet both views. There are times when I choose to use my makeup as a shield helping to boost my confidence when I am taken out of my comfort zone. But by the same token, there are just as many times when I am happy to use makeup as a means of personal expression.

Illusions

The use of colour cosmetics in the form of makeup expertly applied can create the illusion of perfection, detract from areas of the face and body that are less than perfect and draw attention to those areas that hold greater beauty.

Basic rules:

- Dark colours create shade and light colours highlight - generally a shaded area will recede and a highlighted area will become more prominent

- Warm colours may be used to enhance natural warm colouring and/or create a brighter complexion for those with a naturally cool colouring

---

Warm and Cool Colours

Warm colours include those with a yellow base including:

- Gold and bronze
- Lemon and orange
- Beige and conker

Cool colours include those with a blue base including:

- Silver and grey
- Violet and purple
- Pink and magenta

- Browns and reds may be warm or cool depending on the amount of yellow or blue tones added.

- Cool colours may be used to enhance natural cool colouring and/or even out an over-stimulated warm complexion.

Examples of the balancing effects of the use of colour:

- Green counteracts redness. Green has a normalising effect and if applied over areas of high colour will even out the skin tone

- Lilac counteracts yellow. If applied over a sallow skin tone, lilac will lift the complexion

- Yellow counteracts dullness eg under the eyes

- Definition may be created with the use of strong colours to produce harsh lines

- Subtlety may be created with the use of muted colours to produce soft lines

- Shimmer attracts light and emphasises a feature

- A matte effect detracts light and softens a feature

> Youth is enhanced by the use of brightness, definition and shimmer, as these are youthful characteristics. Used on an ageing skin, they will highlight the loss of youthful characteristics. As ageing is accompanied by a softening of features this should be reflected in the application of makeup.

Makeup as a Theory

Bearing in mind the theories associated with beauty and symmetry and the desire to appear *of one's hour* for as long as possible, makeup is used to enhance face shape and skin tone, cheek, eye and lip beauty through skilful blending of light and shade and careful layering.

> Applying concealers and/or foundations with a brush allows for the layering of product providing the potential for better coverage and colour correction.

Makeup as an Art

Makeup lends itself to the creation as well as the interpretation of the new styles that accompany each era. The theories and rules surrounding make-up can be broken in favour of innovation and imagination.

> When it comes to fashion - one person's beauty is another person's ugly.

For many women the world over, their bag of makeup is as important as their wardrobe; they would no more go out with a naked face as with a naked body.

Modern Makeup

The development of the health and beauty industry during the last century has resulted in a merry go round that shows no sign of slowing down. The first few years of the new century still held on to earlier beauty ideals when feminine beauty was associated with childlike delicacy. The Victorian style was very much still in evidence, with floor length dresses and long hair ornately dressed. Cleanliness was next to godliness and the use of makeup frowned upon. Awareness of the toxic nature of the lead-based makeup products used in the past put paid to their use and coloured makeup was very much associated with prostitutes and show girls.

> Powder compacts started to appear at the beginning of the century with small compartments for both rouge and loose powder. Cream rouge was applied under a layer of powder in the quest for a discreet and natural peaches and cream complexion. Whilst the use of makeup was certainly practised it was not readily admitted to.

The suffragette movement saw women taking greater control, with some going as far as to openly wear red lipstick as a means of rebellious expression. This in turn led to the 1920s beauty rush with plucked eyebrows, and pale faces enhanced with reddened lips and cheeks.

Females took on male characteristics both physically and emotionally as the move to liberation began. The introduction of disposable feminine hygiene gave women a freedom that previous bulky sanitary materials had not allowed and so dresses became shorter and more streamlined and attitudes towards beauty changed.

Hairstyles matched the styles of the clothes as the trend for shorter and sleeker took hold. The sexuality of Jean Harlow, Clara Bow and Mae West contrasted with the mysterious, almost androgynous Greta Garbo and Marlene Dietrich. Movie stars showcased the latest fashions as behind the scenes the likes of Coco Chanel, Helena Rubinstein and Elizabeth Arden led the way.

> Nails started to take centre stage with the introduction of high gloss enamels. Nails that had previously been buffed with paste and chamois leather were now lacquered red in the latest style of leaving the half moon crescent shape free.

In the 1930s the Production Code was enforced on Hollywood, which put an end to overt sexuality in films. A more wholesome beauty role model emerged, more traditionally feminine, realistic and achievable. Skirts became once again longer with less emphasis being placed on the legs. Sunbathing was popular and a natural healthy tan encouraged. Katherine Hepburn epitomised this image with discreet makeup and classic style. Women were advised to 'match their lip and nail colours' and to follow the 'Beauty Secrets from Bond Street', which was fast becoming the beauty centre of London.

> Max Factor made his name adapting and applying makeup for film with products and techniques that would be eventually made available to everyone.

World War II led to more practical, masculine and utilitarian beauty characterised by strong independent women. Face makeup was used on the legs and trousers started to replace skirts as stockings became difficult to get hold of.

> Where makeup as well as stockings were in short supply, shoe polish or gravy browning was used on the legs with a seam drawn up the centre of the calf with pencil.

Beauty became practical but no less desired. Makeup was seen as being part of the war effort and women were encouraged to look their best to boost the morale of the troops. Lipsticks and nail polishes took on powerful names to reflect the women who bought them rather than the colour.

The end of the war saw Estée Lauder come onto the beauty scene in 1946 in New York, and beauty also made its first appearance at sea as Steiner opened a salon on board the Queen Mary.

> During this time Christian Dior developed the controversial New Look (which had a small waist and full skirts, and was thought to be extravagant with hitherto rationed material), and reintroduced a more feminine beauty ideal. Movie stars such as Vivienne Leigh, Joan Crawford, Bette Davis and Rosalind Russell reigned.

Post war conservative values and utilitarian attitudes began to be replaced with the glamorous housewife image, as women of the 1950s reconnected with feminine and frivolous beauty. Advances in product manufacture and availability coincided with the changing roles of women and demand for makeup increased. The end of rationing saw a boom in makeup production and by the mid 1950s there were in the region of 50 different brands of lipstick available.

> Revlon's glamorous range of matching lipsticks and nail enamels launched in the Fire and Ice campaign saw the end of the previous make-do-and-mend war era.

There was now a choice of what was beautiful. Sex sirens such as Marilyn Monroe and Jayne Mansfield lived alongside the serene and classic beauty of the likes of Grace Kelly. The 'glamorous housewife' was a typical image of the era; the use of makeup became widespread and women were encouraged to look beautiful not only throughout the day and evening but also even as they aged.

> Avon brought affordable makeup and skin care to the masses. Originally known as The California Perfume Company it was founded in 1886 by a door-to-door salesman and changed its name in 1939. Avon was introduced into Britain in 1959. The Avon Lady and her products brought glamour to many housewives.

As lifestyles improved, a new teenage style and culture developed which contrasted with that of their parents. Added pressure was put on the beauty ideal with the introduction of the Miss World beauty pageant along with the first Barbie dolls, as well as the publication of *Playboy* magazine.

The 1960s brought women a sense of freedom that was previously denied to them. The availability of the contraceptive pill, the legalisation of abortions, increasing educational and career opportunities contributed to the changing faces of beauty.

> The 1960s replaced the traditional rosy-red lips of the past with the new look shimmering pastels. Mascara - of the spit and brush variety - was widely used with additional eyelashes drawn on, Twiggy style.

Teenagers abandoned the fashion and beauty rules of the past. There emerged a set of Beautiful People who seemed to hold the key to beauty and success. Twiggy made her name in the Swinging Sixties and Mary Quant introduced her bright, bold makeup colours.

The 1970s was the decade of freedom. The hippy movement at the start of the decade and the punk culture towards the end prompted the affluent societies of the world to experiment to become expressive and creative in their quest for beauty.

Movie stars, whilst still powerful role models for beauty, were losing some of their influence as individual expression and creativity gained more in popularity with product development to match. As affluence and influence increased in the 1970s pale was no longer seen as interesting as brown emerged as being best. Faces and bodies were exposed with little thought or care to as much natural and/or artificial sunlight as possible. Sun beds came into their own, as did the use of silver foil to attract maximum sunlight to the body, whilst oils with the exotic aromas of far off places fried the skin. Travel opened up not only a merging of skin colours but also beauty ideals as different cultures were adopted and adapted to suit the youth of the day.

> I remember the day the new high tech sun bed was delivered to the Mayfair salon I was working in. We all stood around the Tardis style metal box in awe of the magic that this space ship of light could yield.

The 1980s brought with it financial and creative excess and beauty emerged as both victor and victim. The means to achieve the beauty ideals of the day increased with product innovation and accessibility but the pressure to achieve ideal beauty increased as the momentum started by the mass media began to exert its influence.

The health and fitness boom of the 1980s continued to bring music, fashion and beauty together as movie stars and actresses appeared in exercise and music videos not only wearing the latest fashion but providing the canvas for the new beauty looks. It was all about the body beautiful - with of course a beautiful face to match.

Designer labels were everywhere and makeup was the fashion accessory of the moment in much the same way as a designer handbag. Madonna and Kylie made their debuts, with Kylie soon replacing her girl-next-door image with Madonna-like sexiness. Princess Diana played a big part in the beauty of this and the following decade. Like many prominent royals of past centuries, this princess brought with her a style and glamour that had been lacking in the current royal family becoming a global style icon who adorned publications worldwide every time she blinked a beautifully made up eye.

> The 1980s was a time of power. Powerful women initiated the idea of power dressing and makeup became its reflection.

An undercurrent beauty backlash occurred during the next decade for some with the waif like models, actresses and musicians and the start of the size zero craze. Fit and healthy gave way to thin and emaciated. Drugs and rock and roll featured heavily in creating this look and the phrase 'heroin chic' evolved - it portrayed the deprived, but was available only to the privileged. Cosmetic surgery, something rarely discussed and almost never admitted to, became accessible and acceptable. Beauty came with a greater set of demands, all focused on youth. Teenage culture had well and truly taken over and beauty had become all about turning back the hands of time.

> Eco-aware consumers demanded cruelty-free products with natural, organic and ethically-sourced ingredients.

The start of the 21st century came with makeup innovations in the form of mineral makeup and air brushing techniques to compliment the developments in skin care products, which were all about lifting and protecting.

Adornment was taken to a new level with multiple tattoos, piercings, permanent makeup, self-tanning and extensions (hair, nails and eyelashes).

Whilst conscience shopping is contributing to the beauty choices of today, colour, performance and credibility continue to dominate the world of beauty.

As the 21st century develops, it cannot be denied that the makeup merry go round is here to stay. However, whether we like the view enough to stay on for the ride is up to us.

CHAPTER THREE

Touch

Nothing we use or hear or touch can be expressed in
words that equal what we are given by the senses.

Hannah Arendt

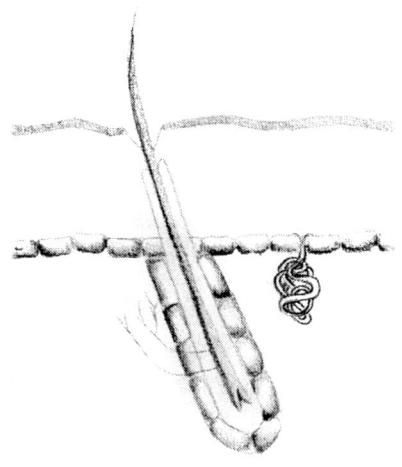

The Science of Touch

The skin's sensory function of touch associated with tactile and thermal feeling is experienced through the skin. Sensory nerves present in the layers of the skin relay messages in the form of electrical impulses along the peripheral nerves to the brain for interpretation. Touch information is passed to the somatosensory cortex in the brain where a map of the whole body is laid out along its surface. The brain in turn interprets what is being felt and where. Touch enables the brain to identify the difference between hot and cold, sharp and soft, pleasure and pain and as the skin forms the largest organ of the body, the associated sense of touch links all parts of the body with the brain providing the ability to nurture, soothe and heal as well as stimulate, invigorate and activate. Touch enhances the other senses creating a sensation that acts as both judge and jury of beauty and a skin that is in good condition further enhances the sense of touch. A thin skin will have heightened feeling, as sensory nerves lie closer to the surface whereas a thickened skin will experience the opposite.

Paraesthesia refers to a loss of tactile sensation that may be of a temporary nature ie the numbness of a limb falling asleep or the pins and needles sensation that is a common result of sustained pressure as well as a symptom of more serious conditions which should be checked out by a doctor if experienced. Reduced or increased skin sensitivity known as tactile hypoaesthesia and tactile hyperaesthesia are also areas of concern as any abnormal response to tactile stimuli can indicate an underlying problem that may need medical attention.

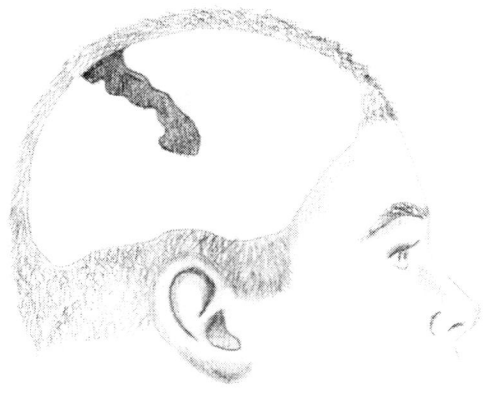

SENSE OF TOUCH

The Art of Touch

Clairsentience, meaning clear touch, refers to one of the extra sensory functions and is associated with the ability to feel vibrational energy without making actual physical contact. This type of touch may be experienced as a barely there sensation anywhere on the body in the form of a soft breeze, a delicate stroke, gentle warmth or a faint coolness and as such is often ignored. Alternatively it may also be experienced by some with much greater impact in the form of a blast of air, a push or shove, extreme heat or excessive cold making it much harder to ignore. Either way, clairsentience is an extra sensory function that requires greater awareness and understanding before it is universally accepted.

Skin has the ability to reflect the beauty of more than just itself.

The general condition of a person can be seen as well as felt. The skin is a showcase for the innermost workings of the body as it reflects the glowing bloom of youth and tracks its fading glory as age, use and abuse take their toll.

Reflexology is the art and science of treating the whole body through an individual part; the skin of the feet, hands and ears are good examples of this theory. Each of these areas of the body provide a unique insight into the working and well being of the whole body through the concept of zones, meridians, chakras and reflex points. The eastern cultures of the world have long believed that the various parts of the body are intrinsically linked and their methods of healing such as acupuncture, shiatsu and reiki have paid tribute to this theory.

However, it wasn't until the late 1800s and early 1900s that western scientists confirmed this as fact, as their knowledge of the nervous system developed, together with a greater understanding of the human form and function. The discovery of the links between the skin and the brain through the peripheral nerves coincided with the experimentation of pain relief with treatment to a part of the body ie reflexology in order to affect the whole body closely following. Quite by accident it was discovered that by applying pressure to one body part it had the effect of helping to block pain in a corresponding area.

It was an American ear, nose and throat surgeon Dr. William Fitzgerald who, in the early 1900s, acknowledged that prior to the use of modern methods of pain relief, his patients would hold tightly onto the operating chair or press their feet firmly onto the floor. He and his contemporaries experimented with the use of gadgets such as pegs and elastic bands as well as manual pressure applied firmly to the ends of the digits whilst operating on other areas and explored the concept of 10 longitudinal zones – five on each side of body linked to each toe, thumb and finger.

It was found that if pressure was applied anywhere within a zone it had the potential to have an effect on any corresponding area of the same zone. As the hands and indeed the feet offered the easiest access to manipulation further experimentation led to the discovery that the organs of the body could be mapped out on palms of the hands and the soles of the feet as pressure in certain areas appeared to relieve pain in corresponding organs. A physiotherapist of the time, Eunice Ingham, devoted her whole adult life to this theory adding a form of therapeutic massage to replace the gadgets and pressure techniques previously used by incorporating alternate pressure movements known as finger/thumb walking. The resulting treatment was reflexology – treatment of the whole body through a part.

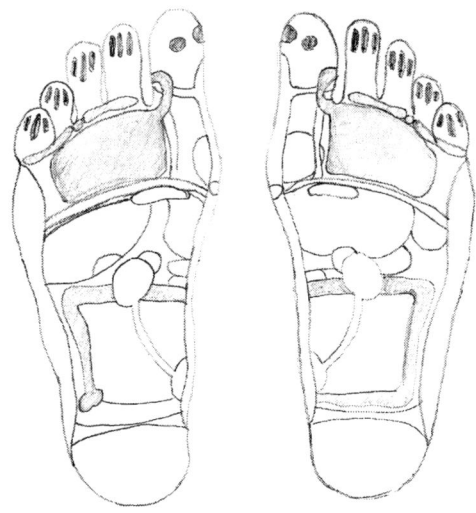

REFLEXOLOGY CHART

Skin Facts – The Physical Skin

The skin is composed of two main parts – the uppermost **epidermis** and the underlying **dermis**. The epidermis consists of cells arranged in layers that constantly push themselves up to the surface as part of the renewal process known as **mitosis**. The living cells gradually die off as they reach the surface and are shed from the body in a natural process known as **desquamation**. The hair and nails develop from the living cells, gradually dying off as they also renew through the same process of mitosis, pushing their way to the surface forming the strands of hair that cover various parts of the body and the hard plates of nail that protect the ends of the fingers, thumbs and toes.

> The skin, hair and nails are collectively known as the integumentary system of the body offering a protective covering that may be likened to a living suit of armour.

The inherent colour of the skin is determined in the epidermis with the formation of the natural pigment known as **melanin**. The cells that produce melanin are further stimulated by ultra violet light and activated to produce the varying amounts of colour associated with natural tanning.

The underlying dermis is formed from a variety of protein fibres including **collagen** and **elastin** responsible for the youthfulness and elasticity associated with young skin.

Ageing sees a deterioration in these fibres that in turn contributes to the changes experienced in texture and loss of tone. Sweat is produced in the dermis contributing to the regulation of body temperature and its production is activated by emotional stress as well as changes in the internal environment of the physical body. The formation of goose pimples on the surface of the skin works in opposition to the production of sweat in a quest to maintain correct body temperature but like sweat they are also produced as a result of emotional stimulus. In addition, the skin's natural oil known as **sebum** is also produced within the dermis contributing to the hydration levels of the skin, hair and nails.

The fat deposits of the body lie directly below the dermis in an area known as the **hypodermis** or **subcutaneous layer**. The fat deposits form **adipose tissue** essential for insulation and added protection but detrimental if excessive due to the pressure exerted on the heart to maintain a constant blood supply to all areas.

The surface of the skin has a natural covering known as the acid mantle which is comprised of a small amount of dead skin cells, sweat and sebum offering a degree of external protection. When the acid mantle is intact the skin feels and appears neither dry and taut nor oily and shiny.

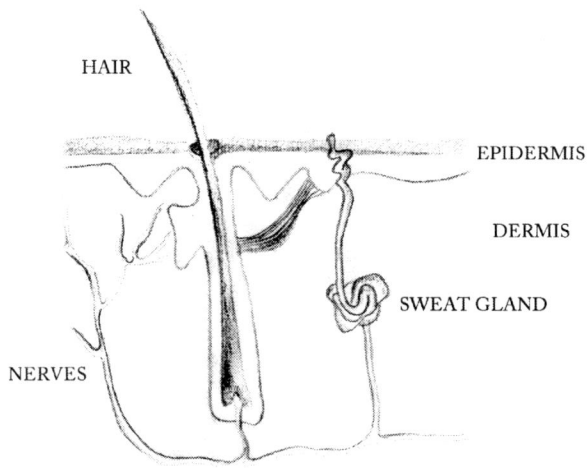

Skin Facts – The Emotional Skin

The skin is an emotional organ as well as physical one with the ability to express a number of emotions thus acting as a barometer for our innermost feelings. In fact the **integumentary** system as a whole, including the skin, hair and nails, is highly responsive capable of communicating a whole range of strong emotions all of which add to the complete beauty picture:

- The skin blushes pink with embarrassment and flushes red with anger.

- Its colour drains with shock and mottles with emotional confusion.

- Hairs stand on end as heartfelt passion forces the tiny muscles of the skin to contract forming the characteristic goose bumps.

- Bitten down nails and cuticles together with thinning hair from constant tugging, pulling or twisting accompany a nervous or stressed disposition.

- Reflexologists also subscribe to the concept that certain external skin and nail conditions are signs of internal emotion turmoil including:

  o Hard skin denoting the need for emotional protection as well as offering physical protection of a part.

  o Peeling skin signalling the release of old emotions.

  o Puffiness relating to stagnation of emotions and an overloaded of feelings.

  o Rough areas of skin relating to a person experiencing a tough time emotionally.

  o Cracked skin suggesting a splitting of feelings and of emotions being torn apart.

o   Tautness of skin resulting from feeling 'strung up' and 'stressed out'.

o   Nails that lift, demonstrating a 'head in clouds' attitude whilst nails that curve downwards display a person's need to 'keep their feet on the ground'.

In addition to portraying an emotion through the skin, it is also possible to be emotionally 'touched' by an action or deed, object or subject. This usually refers to something that is heartfelt and positive such as affection, sympathy, and empathy and signifies warmth and inclusion. Strong emotions may also linger in the air even after the feelings have been expressed and the resulting atmosphere felt by a third party, as in the phrase 'you could cut the air with a knife' despite having no previous involvement.

Skin Facts – The Spiritual Skin

A person's **aura** describes the energy field that is the physical body and that which surrounds it and is believed to form a link between the physical, emotional and the spiritual personae. The aura consists of seven layers or bodies that interconnect with the chakras reflecting and responding to the frequencies and vibrations associated with the colours present in light and as such have the potential to be seen (although not always in their entirety) and felt.

- The physical body reflects the human form.
- The etheric body reflects the physical body.
- The astral body reflects emotions.
- The lower mental body reflects thought patterns.
- The higher mental body reflects intuition.
- The causal body reflects the cause for current life together with a record of all past lives.
- The bodiless body reflects a person's true essence or spirit.

Skin Beauty

The perfect skin is said to be clear in appearance and even in texture.

A youthful skin may be likened to a ripe plum whilst an ageing skin takes on the characteristics of a shrivelled prune. The ripe plum represents youth, lustre and fertility ie being of one's hour. Conversely, the prune is synonymous with loss – loss of youth, loss of lustre and loss of fertility. For most, the former symbolises beauty whilst the latter has forfeited its beauty.

Perfect head hair may be straight, wavy or curly but must be manageable. It may be of any colour other than grey with blonde taking favour for many. Body hair comes and goes with fashion and fads either hiding the underlying areas of skin or bearing them in all of their glory.

Perfect nails should appear pink in colour up to the tip, which should be a clear, bright white. The length and shape of nails fluctuate with fashion but should ideally reflect the shape of the base, be even on both hands with cuticles that are neatly eased back to show perfect, pearly half moon shapes.

> It is commonly believed that the larger the half moon appears the higher a person's breeding.

The skin has the ability to reflect inner beauty and provide outer beauty.

From time immemorial humans have attempted to either enhance or disguise their skin in order to lead or follow the beauty ideals of their day and in doing so make an individual or collective mark on beauty history. Throughout history the skin, hair and nails have also proved to be ideal canvasses on which to demonstrate creativity, skill and art which every culture and era has made use of in one form or another eg

- **Painting** – colour plays an important role in creating a beauty illusion with the skilful art of makeup.
- **Scarring** – is used by some cultures to as a means of 'branding' creating a look that conforms to a certain beauty ideal.
- **Tattooing** – reflects an added value beauty of personal creativity.
- **Piercing** – adorns and enhances natural beauty subject to personal standards.

- **Cutting** – surgery to produce conformity of beauty and/or youth.

- **Replacing** – adding to or taking away in order to create an ideal beauty.

From painting through to replacing and everything in between the skin remains a focal point for the attainment of beauty that may at first glance appear to be only skin deep, yet beneath its exterior lies an emotional and spiritual core.

Skin Power

Physically the skin has the power to withstand a great deal in its quest to protect the vital inner organs of the body. Acting like a living suit of armour, it resists invasion from harmful substances, endures the changes in weather and temperature extremes, and survives the stretch of weight gain and pregnancy as well as adding to a person's unique and individual powers of attraction. Through touch, the skin has the power to give and receive the extremes of human emotion from love and hate through to kill or cure and it is generally accepted that the person who is performing the touch is the one who holds the greater power. A person who is referred to as being a 'soft touch' is commonly regarded as one who has minimal power in much the same way as someone who has 'lost their touch' is seen as being inferior to those who have not.

The Language of The Skin

Haptic communication refers to the varying messages that touch is able to communicate between people and may be characterised as being:

- **Functional** referring to touch that is supportive and helpful, eg a guiding hand.

- **Social** relating to polite touching that is respectful and mindful. A handshake is a prime example.

- **Platonic** associated with touch that conveys feelings of warmth and friendship eg a kiss on the cheek (from friendship discussed by the Greek philosopher Plato)

- **Intimate** referring to the touch that signals unconditional loving care, eg a mother's touch.

- **Sexual** associated with touch that initiates a state of arousal.

As with all methods of communication there exists cultural, social and personal boundaries with barriers that need to be defined and agreed before touch can take place in order to avoid possible misinterpretation and offence.

> Tactile sign language is a communication tool used by both the deaf and blind in the form of finger spelling, Braille etc.

Skin Care

The skin, as the largest organ of the body, has many important functions including protection of the underlying bones, muscles and organs, regulation of body temperature through the production of sweat and the action of goose bumps, production of sebum (the skin's natural oil) and vitamin D (produced in sunlight helping the body store calcium vital for healthy bones and teeth), and as a sensory organ contributes to keeping the brain informed of tactile and thermal sensations.

The skin has a complex structure that undergoes a constant renewal process throughout life speeding up in childhood whilst slowing down with age. With its accompanying hair and nails it is reliant on care and attention and whilst the skin care products used go a long way in supporting its functions, knowledge and understanding is the key to its welfare.

The skin is essentially made up of protein fibres that form many layers. This layering effect gives the skin its strength, resilience, elasticity and ultimately its beauty. It comes in a variety of shades due to the hereditary distribution of colour pigment melanin, which offers further protection to the inner body and the potential for enhanced beauty to the outer body. Hair and nails develop and grow from within the skin protruding as dead, hardened structures that offer additional protection to sensitive areas of the body as well as providing further scope for external beauty. Hair growth, colour and lustre have long been associated with fertility and piety whilst nails offer a reflection of lifestyle and both are constant fashion victims.

Directly below the skin lies fatty tissue providing the body with insulation, an extra energy source as well as shape. At puberty hormones inform the female body to begin to store the excess fat around the hip and thigh area of the body whilst in males, hormones direct the fat to be stored around the abdomen thus changing the shape of a young male and female as they enter adulthood and beyond. Muscles bulk up in males and females develop breasts and, as the body takes on more of these secondary sexual characteristics, the skin accommodates the changes enhancing the developing sexuality and beauty.

Meanwhile, throughout a person's life the skin, hair and nails are constantly undergoing a state of renewal and change as surface cells die and are shed, many millions more are getting ready to take their place. A whole network of cellular activity occurs below the surface of the skin as new cells form fresh layers which in turn push their way up to the surface changing their shape and action as they contribute to each ascending layer.

Sebum is produced within these layers contributing to the lustre of the skin and hair whilst a complex blood supply helps to regulate body temperature as well as give the skin and nails their characteristic healthy bloom.

At puberty apocrine sweat glands present in the skin and found amongst the genital, breast and underarm areas of the body are activated producing sweat that as it breaks down is responsible for our individual body odour. This sweat as opposed to the sweat produced in the rest of the body by eccrine sweat glands, which is essentially associated with temperature control, is designed to make us sexually attractive.

As the skin, hair and nails renew they feed off everything that is put into the body – from the air we breathe to the food and water that we eat and drink even to the thoughts we think, offering a reflection of a person's physical effectiveness and emotional state at each and every stage of their existence. In addition to this, the skin, hair and nails respond to everything that is put onto them offering a living suit of armour to the precious organs lying below and whilst much may be done to enhance and embellish them, nothing can stop the passage of time and its debilitating effects on their appearance.

> Free radicals are the by product of energy production eg pollution, sunlight, cellular activity etc. and are ultimately responsible for the ageing process. Premature ageing occurs as a result of over exposure to free radicals.

In order to reproduce, skin cells rely on energy production and the by product of this energy production is what is ultimately responsible for the signs of ageing as skin, hair and nails lose their lustre and bloom forming the telltale signs of ageing. External energy production in the form of sunlight and pollution adds to their gradual deterioration and premature ageing and further deterioration occurs if exposure is too great and unprotected. Whilst the skin, hair and nails care for the internal organs by forming a protective covering that we all too often take for granted, they also rely heavily on the continual care of the rest of the body to maintain their structure, functions and ultimately, their beauty.

Care of the skin follows a set of golden rules that may be applied to the body as a whole and are associated with the four Rs: release, replenish, reaction and respond:

Release

The constant renewal process known as mitosis by which the skin cells develop relies on energy production. Waste products accompany the production of energy and need to be constantly released. Urine contains the waste products of cellular energy production whilst faeces contain the waste products of digestion and calls of nature should be heeded for the skin to benefit. Failure to do so results in congested skin, prone to problems.

Cellular waste is picked up by the lymphatic system, which works closely with blood circulation and consists of a set of vessels for transportation, strategically placed nodes for filtration and ducts to connect it with veins. The lymphatic system produces cells that are able to engulf harmless substances and destroy them as part of the body's immune functions.

Replenish

Skin cells rely on nutrients to maintain their structure and function. Water, proteins, carbohydrates, fats, vitamins and minerals are all necessary components of effective cell renewal and need to be regularly replenished. A regular, stable diet is the basic internal requirement of skin maintenance together with the sensible application of products to service its exterior.

Food Facts

Water makes up 70% of an average cell. Drinking water and eating foods with a high water content keeps the water levels in cells topped up.

The dermis contains protein fibres in the form of collagen and elastin contributing to the youthfulness and elasticity of skin. Food rich in protein are needed for the growth and repair of skin cells.

Carbohydrates are needed for skin cells to produce energy. Therefore foods containing slow releasing carbohydrates provide the skin with the means to function effectively throughout each day.

Fat is stored in the hypodermis providing vital insulation and cushioning. Unsaturated fats provide a healthier option than saturated animal fats.

Vitamins and minerals are necessary requirements enabling the skin to maintain its protective functions as well as aid in fighting free radical attack.

Reaction

Skin cells require a state of homeostasis or equilibrium in order to maintain their well being and beauty thereby a stimulating reaction needs to be counteracted by a calming response. Maintaining a balance between rest and activity is vital for the skin, which with age is quicker to display the price of fatigue and increasingly slower to demonstrate the signs associated with rest.

> Cellular renewal relies on equal amounts of stimulation for the transportation of nutrients to each cell and waste products away from each cell and peace, quiet and calm in order to carry out its specific functions.

Respond

The key to healthy and beautiful skin is to take note of its demands and in doing so ensure that its physical, emotional and spiritual needs are taken care of. It really is that straightforward!

> Chinese facial analysis aims to make a diagnosis of the body through the scrutiny of the face and its features.

Skin Care Specifics

Children's skin up to puberty maintains a balanced function, which is reflected in its natural beauty. Puberty and the subsequent life cycles associated with pregnancy and menopause (andropause in males) together with physical, emotional and spiritual stress initiate a set of reactions that can cause the skin to change resulting in the problems associated with congestion, sensitivity, dehydration and premature ageing. As a result, the skin will demand extra care, telling us exactly what it needs and when. Whilst this may seem like a foreign language, interpretation and action is not as difficult as it may at first appear:

Skin types may be classified as being:

- **Normal** – usually associated with a young prepubescent skin or one with no apparent problems
- **Oily** – oversecretion of the skin's natural oil sebum will be seen as a shiny surface and be accompanied with varying degrees of congestion. Often associated with puberty it is compounded by poor diet, lack of or incorrect skin care and certain types of medication and drugs
- **Dry** – underproduction of the skin's natural oil sebum will be seen as a dull, flaky surface and be accompanied by varying degrees of tautness. Often associated with aging, it may also be a direct result of

poor diet, lack of or incorrect skin care, over exposure to UV light, illness, medication and drugs

- **Combination** – the skin will often demonstrate a combination of types ie oily along the centre T zone where there is a greater number of sebum producing glands and normal or drier cheeks and neck. This skin type is perhaps the most common of all and one of the most confusing to treat

All skin types respond well to a morning and evening routine of cleansing, toning and moisturising:
- Cleansing – choose oil free washes for oily skins, lotions for normal and creams for dry
- Toning – choose astringents for oily skins eg witch hazel, fresheners for normal eg orange flower water and hydrators for dry eg rose water
- Moisturising – choose anti bacterial lotions for oily skin, lotions for normal and creams for dry

In addition to the main skin types there are also classifications of skin problems that may accompany any of the above in the form of:

Congestion resulting in open, blocked and enlarged pores, blemishes in the form of papules, pustules and blackheads and may be external and/or internal:

- External congestion refers to excess sebum coating the surface of the skin in which dead skin cells, dirt, dust and makeup become stuck

- Internal congestion refers to inefficient removal of cellular waste in localised areas

Congestion responds well to both external and internal treatment:

- External exfoliation helps to clear surface congestion
- Increased water intake helps to flush out internal congestion

Sensitivity resulting in areas of heightened feeling and colour and often accompanies a pale, thin and see-through skin that is prone to allergies and eczema

Sensitivity responds well to gentle treatment and mild products.

Sensitivity tests are recommended prior to the use of a new product to ensure compatibility.

Dehydration resulting in skin that ages prematurely as skin cells are deprived of the water they need to function effectively. Lines and wrinkles are common signs of a dehydrated skin.

To check for dehydration: pinch the skin on the back of the hand so that it tents up. Hold the skin for a few seconds before releasing it. Skin should quickly return to normal. If this is not the case and the skin is slow to return to normal it will be an indication of dehydration.

To remedy dehydration: increase fluid intake in the form of still water at room temperature (easiest for the body to absorb) and ensure foods are introduced into the diet that contain water eg fruit and vegetables.

Skin beauty will ultimately be reflected in skin care.

Thoughts and Theories

What we think of our skin and how we feel about it is as important to its beauty as how we care for it.

There are many myths and misconceptions surrounding the attainment of the body beautiful, which often cloud the judgment and hinder the acceptance of the natural beauty cycles of life leading to dissatisfaction and with it the desire to make changes.

Inherent factors are ignored in favour of fashion and trend and a growing 'Jim'll fix it' quick fix culture threatens to produce clones of a single moment in the beauty timeline. However, bodies come in all shapes and sizes and no two bodies are the same and yet despite this fact there is the desire to seek that which we are not or are no longer.

Somatotypes: Dr. William Sheldon (1898-1977) an American psychologist developed a system of three body types with specific characteristics:

- Ectomorph refers to a body type that is long limbed, slim, lean and angular with little body fat or muscle bulk and does not gain weight easily
- Mesomorph refers to a body type that is broad, muscular and athletic and has a tendency to gain weight slowly over time
- Endomorph refers to a body type that is short, curvaceous, stocky and plump with a tendency to gain weight easily

Most people are predominantly of one particular body type but will share some characteristics of the others; these characteristics are inherited and as such are non transferable.

Pain versus Gain

*Exercise is the deliberate and planned movement of
the human frame, accompanied by breathlessness
for the sake of health and fitness.*
Hieronymus Mercurialis (1530-1601)

It was the popular exercise culture, of the 1970/80s that
coined the now infamous phrase of 'no pain, no gain'. This
gave rise to a school of thought that believed the body and
mind needed to undergo a certain amount of suffering in
order to achieve a beauty ideal. The more you suffered, the
greater the gain.

This was hardly a new way of thinking, but the developing
world was replacing the tortuous methods of Chinese foot
binding, tribal neck stretching and figure-changing corsetry
with modern, no less painful versions. Aerobic exercising
swept through the world promising the perfection of a movie
star body if you could just bear to 'feel the burn'. Dressed in
unforgiving Lycra, nations of men as well as women of all ages
and sizes took to the gym in hot and painful pursuit of the
body beautiful with little or no regard to body structure and
type or levels of health and fitness.

What resulted was a great deal of pain but very little gain
as drained and dehydrated bodies were brought to their knees

by pounding hearts, strained lungs and overworked muscles, bones and joints.

As the potential for physical stress increased, so did the mental strain of having to cope with the repeated failure of the body to respond in the imagined way. Logic lost its reason as another branch of the beauty industry gained its own momentum, adding greater pressure to the attainment of a perfect beauty.

> Through the nervous system, the body offers a foolproof means to maintaining its overall wellbeing safely and effectively. The varying degrees of pain the body is capable of feeling provides a way of determining its value and the idea that pain equals gain is not usually correct. In physiological terms, pain is the body's way of alerting the recipient to the fact that enough is enough and the pain causing activity should be stopped.

Physical activity is a necessary component of a healthy life style but needs to be approached with care and attention paid to the specific needs of an individual with regards to age, weight, body type, sex and health and fitness levels.

> The need for exercise was identified as being an essential part of health as far back as 400 years before the birth of Christ. Hippocrates, the ancient Greek physician and father of medicine is reported to have stated that "If we could give every individual the right amount of nourishment and exercise, not too little and not too much, we would have found the safest way to health."

In the past, exercise has been approached with a variety of different mindsets and although physicians have long agreed that a modicum of physical activity is a basic requirement of health, exercising as we know it today was slow to develop.

> Aulus Cornelius Celsus (c 25-50BC) an eminent encyclopaedist, described in his work *De Medicina* "Take exercise for whilst inaction weakens the body, work strengthens it; the former brings on premature ageing, the latter prolongs youth."

Despite evidence to the contrary it was once thought that weight training slowed down athletes and that endurance training was not good for the heart. Exercise was deemed unhealthy for women and too strenuous for the elderly. However, the decreasing fitness levels of young men entering the forces in the 1950s demonstrated the loss of physical health that was accompanying the increasing standards of living. Labour saving devices were drastically reducing the amount of daily physical activity for many people and resulting health studies initiated the need for individuals to take exercise to compensate.

This led to the popularity of gyms and the introduction of home gym equipment. Treadmills, static bikes and rowers were added to the growing number of electrical appliances within many homes and an exercise boom followed, culminating in the aerobics revolution that saw groups of like minded, if not always like-bodied people strut their stuff to the Seventies' and Eighties' beat for all their worth.

> Prior to the development of the exercise and spa industries and their accompanying qualifications, beauty therapists were trained to give exercise lessons. Many salons incorporated a small gym, which contained such antiquities as vibrating body belts, wooden pummelling machines as well as a variety of basic weights, bands and balls. Exercise routines would be softer versions of the army boot camp directives and instruction given on a one to one basis prior to the application of a heat and/or massage treatment.

What ultimately developed from the hype was an industry that through research and standardisation has gained in knowledge and stature providing a range of exercise activities to suit everyone that aim to take into account the individual and very different inherent physical characteristics and whilst exercising no longer claims to give you Jane Fonda's body, it does claim to make the most of what you've got which may just prove to be the answer to perfect beauty – or is it?

> For general health and fitness it is recommended that 30 minutes a day is spent in some form of exercise and it is wise to alternate the type and level to allow for rest and recuperation. Studies have also shown that it is as important to exercise the mind; the phrase 'Use it or lose it' refers to the brain as well as the body.

Trial and Tribulation

The constant quest to achieve and preserve body beauty perfection has inevitably brought with it numerous trials that history demonstrates have not been without error as well as a whole host of tribulations that have at times resulted in extremes of mental and physical suffering.

Destruction, disfigurement and even death through product poisoning, surgery mistakes and misdemeanours as well as myriad eating phobias and disorders can all stake a claim in the age-old search for body beauty.

The advancements in science and technology have as much to answer for in the pursuit of perfection as the beauty and advertising industries have in creating supply and demand. However, as the medical profession progressed through the 19th and 20th centuries so did the development and use of electrical machinery. Aimed primarily at treating specific medical problems, the machines were soon found to have secondary positive effects associated with skin and body care. This led to adaptations of such machines being made for use within the beauty industry including:

Mechanical massage machines:

- **Gyratory massagers** eg G5, an electrically powered massage machine that uses a variety of different attachments to simulate manual massage with the potential for greater depth and pressure. Used on the body as an aid to slimming.

> In the late 1970s many Arab ladies visited London with their wealthy husbands and sought treatments in salons. G5 proved to be a particularly popular treatment in pummelling away the excesses of their good and plentiful lives.

- **Audio sonic vibrator:** an electromagnetic hand held massage machine producing sound waves that vibrate deep into the underlying tissue of the body. This has a relaxing effect at a deep level without stimulating the surface skin.

- **Vacuum suction:** a vacuum pump driven by an electric motor to create a static or intermittent suction. Vacuum suction produces a gently stimulating action, which used on the face plumps up skin tissue reducing the signs of ageing and is used as an aid to slimming on the body.

> Vacuum suction should not be mistaken for liposuction, which is a surgical procedure removing excess fat from specific areas of the body.

- **Microdermabrasion:** incorporates the use of a compressor to draw up air through a tube, which causes micro crystals placed at the opposite end to be sucked towards an applicator probe. Placed onto the skin the micro crystals have the effect of gently breaking down the surface skin cells, which are then removed by suction. Also known as a skin peeling treatment.

Electrotherapy machines:

- **High frequency:** an alternating or oscillating electrical current that may be applied directly or indirectly through the use of glass electrodes and manual massage. Direct high frequency aids in the treatment of acne and associated problems whilst indirect high frequency provides an anti-ageing effect.

> Direct high frequency was once a popular hair treatment performed in hair salons. Glass comb or bulb electrodes were used to stimulate hair growth in the never-ending quest to aid hair loss and balding.

- **Galvanic:** a smooth flowing, uninterrupted direct electrical current applied to the skin via electrodes. Used with both a negative polarity for an alkaline and destructive effect known as desincrustation, which is deep cleansing and stimulating, and a positive polarity, which is soothing and calming having the effect of restoring the skin's natural acid pH and known as iontophoresis. Used on the face its aids skin problems and on the body it helps eliminate the telltale signs of cellulite.

> Popular electrical treatments are often referred to by their brand or manufacturer's names rather than the type of electrical current they use adding to the confusion surrounding the use of electrical machinery.

- **Faradic:** an alternating low frequency, surged and interrupted direct electrical current passes through pads which are strategically placed over muscles to effect an isometric contraction ie exercising with activity. Used to strengthen and tone muscles improving body shape and contour.

Body faradic is a popular home treatment with pads being inserted into special belts or shorts for treatment of the abdomen, hips and thighs. Facial faradic for home use is also popular and incorporates sticky pads that are placed over specific muscles. Marketed as having the benefits of exercise without the hard work.

- **Micro current**: a modified direct current interrupted at low frequencies used with a variety of electrodes as a gentle and effective way of re-educating motor nerves to improve muscle function.

Micro current facials are marketed as 'non surgical facelifts'.

- **Epilation**: the permanent removal of hair and may be applied in three ways via the use of a fine needle inserted into the hair follicle. The *galvanic* method incorporates a direct current producing a chemical reaction. The *diathermy* method uses a high frequency alternating current that produces heat. The *blend* method combines diathermy and galvanic to produce a more effective result.

Electrolysis is a term commonly used to describe permanent hair removal. Electrolysis in fact refers to the chemical reaction that occurs during galvanic epilation.

Heat producing machines:

- **Wax pots**: use electricity to heat the contents which can include warm or hot wax for depilation (semi permanent methods of hair removal) or paraffin wax for nourishing body treatments

Before the introduction of thermostatically controlled wax pots salons would use double ring burners and saucepans and manually test the temperature of the wax. Hot wax would be applied with wooden spoons and, once removed, was reheated in a second pot before being strained through a metal sieve prior to its next application. Waxes would be delivered to the salons in massive slabs, which required a hammer and chisel to cut through.

- **Steamers**: use electricity to heat water to produce steam. Steam may be used to warm the skin and underlying tissue offering a relaxing treatment for the whole body, which may be used for isolated areas to treat skin congestion.

Essential oils may be added to steaming units infusing the steam with their specific properties providing greater value to the steaming experience.

- **Infra red**: uses infra-red rays to heat the superficial tissue for a relaxing and soothing effect. Commonly used as a pre-massage treatment for maximum relaxation.

- **Ultra violet**: sun tanning equipment use high levels of artificial UVA rays together with some UVB rays within tubes or lamps to stimulate the production of the skin's natural colour pigment known as melanin.

The 1970s saw the introduction of sun beds in salons which were met with much excitement as with the introduction of spray tanning of more recent years.

- **Laser and IPL (intense pulsed light):** the use of high-energy beams of light was introduced in the 1990s to treat skin problems associated with acne, sun damage, thread and varicose veins and more recently the removal of hair.

Nowadays, the use of such machines is regulated and should not be applied by anyone other than someone who has been correctly trained, suitably qualified, certificated and who has up to date insurance. Anyone seeking such treatments should expect to have a consultation whereby treatment choice and application is fully explained and any contraindications (reasons for not being able to have the treatment) checked and contra actions (possible after effects) advised upon. Only then do these treatments become effective and safe in providing a suitable option in the beauty quest.

> Electrical treatments for home use should come with a cautionary health warning as they can become, for some addictive. Excessive use of any treatment may result in skin damage rather than skin care eg overuse of sun beds.

Needle or Knife?

Whilst the use of electrical machines in the quest for the face and body beautiful has become a recognised part of the beauty industry there has been a growing sideline of surgical procedures that offer quicker, better and longer lasting results, but despite the hype, still come at some considerable cost.

These procedures involve going under the needle or knife and the cost may be physical and emotional as well as financial.

The desire to conform to an idealistic beauty image as well as to turn back the hands of time dates back to antiquity. The ancient Greeks coined the phrase plastic surgery from their word *plastikos* meaning to 'mould or shape' and it has been used in a variety of ways by many ancient cultures either to enhance their dead so that they would be recognised in the afterlife, repair structures such as noses and ears damaged as a result of punishment or battle injuries and even in some cases to correct areas of the body seen to be wanting with much the same attitude as in today's society.

Aulus Cornelius Celsus also described plastic surgery of the face using skin from other parts of the body.

However, the early procedures were crude and fraught with problems associated with the extreme pain of surgery without anaesthetics and the life threatening infections that inevitably followed, but with the gradual advancements in science and technology together with increased knowledge of the human function and form a number of innovations have evolved over the past century to become an integral part of the beauty world including cosmetic surgery, injectable and dermal fillers.

Cosmetic or aesthetic plastic surgery takes its origins from reconstructive surgery, which was developed to correct the structure and function of areas of the body that had been impaired by burns, injury or congenital abnormalities. In contrast, cosmetic surgery was developed for enhancement, augmentation and reduction of body parts to meet the beauty ideals of the day.

> The first facelifts were performed in the early 1900s and involved simply making an incision, pulling back the skin, removing any excess before closing up the incision. Today's facelifts now involve repositioning the superficial musculoaponeurotic system (SMAS), which basically means that the skin and underlying muscles and nerves are repositioned to provide a more natural looking result.

A plastic surgeon may be found to perform cosmetic surgery on most every part of the body with new innovations occurring almost daily as the need to alter the human form becomes as desirable and accessible as donning a new pair of shoes.

> The more bizarre cosmetic procedures include toe surgery to improve toe cleavage to meet the demands of a perceived shoe fashion, and Brazilian buttock augmentation to create a shape that is inherent in certain body types and desirable in others.

Injectable and dermal fillers have been around for over a century with physicians developing ways to restore volume and structure to ageing skin. The introduction of syringes made this a possibility, and experimentation saw the use of fillers such as paraffin, silicone and collagen and more recently botox, hyaluronic acid and fat.

Glossary of Terms

- **Paraffin** was one of the early fillers but its use was limited and soon rejected for other alternatives
- **Silicones** are an inactive synthetic compound that have been widely used but not without problems especially those associated with leakage
- **Collagen** is a naturally occurring protein present in humans and animals and is responsible for the plumpness of cells associated with youth. Collagen from cows and pigs' skin has been used for injectable fillers
- **Botox** or botulinum toxin is a protein produced by a bacterium. When injected into the body it has the effect of blocking nerve impulses and has found uses in the treatment of excessive blinking (blepharospasm), squints (strabismus), excessive sweating (hyperhidrosis) and muscle pain in addition to the reduction of the expression lines and wrinkles associated with the use of facial muscles that accompanies the ageing process
- **Hyaluronic acid** is a natural substance present in the body that retains water and strengthens the collagen and elastin protein bonds adding volume to the skin's surface. It may be produced from a bacterium as well as synthetically to be used as injectable fillers
- **Fat** harvested from different areas of the body eg hips and thighs may be used as fillers for other areas eg face

- **Stem cell technology** is exploring the possibility of using these special cells produced in the body that are capable of not only reproducing themselves but also with the ability to develop into specific types of cells with the view to improvement

All cosmetic applications are temporary, invasive (some more than others) and costly and not without the potential for problems. Not only do mistakes occur, but also the result may not be what was expected, often the cause of further heartache. The resulting new physical identity may prove to be at odds with a person's emotional identity and many cases see that person changing their mind about the alterations they have sought. The part of the body may not feel the same nor have the same sense of feeling and instead of remaining a natural part of the whole body it takes on almost alien characteristics that may be difficult to come to terms with. In the case of treatment as an anti ageing tool, nothing can stop the passage of time and whilst it continues to progress forward so too will the natural ageing process and although it may be possible to slow it down, acceptance of the inevitable cannot ultimately be denied. Cosmetic surgery has become for some an acceptable way of achieving and maintaining beauty longevity and is thought to hold the key to the beauty of the future.

But does this really answer all of the needs of beauty or does it just pay tribute to its superficial layers confirming that beauty is indeed merely skin deep?

CHAPTER FOUR

Smell

It is a golden maxim to cultivate the garden for
the nose, and the eyes will take care of themselves.
Robert Louis Stevenson

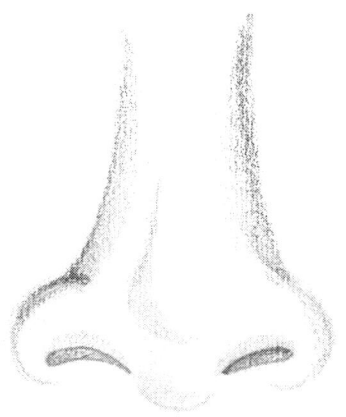

The Sense of Smell

The sensory function associated with the ability of the nose to detect odour is known as **olfaction**. As odour gases in the air are breathed into the body special olfactory cells at the back of the nose pass the information to the brain via the first cranial, olfactory, nerves. The odour information is processed low down in the prefrontal lobe of the brain in the **limbic centre** which interprets the aromas. The limbic area of the brain is also responsible for the interpretation of taste, which is closely linked to the sense of smell. It also acts as a memory store: the sensory functions associated with smell and taste can evoke instantaneous and powerful memories.

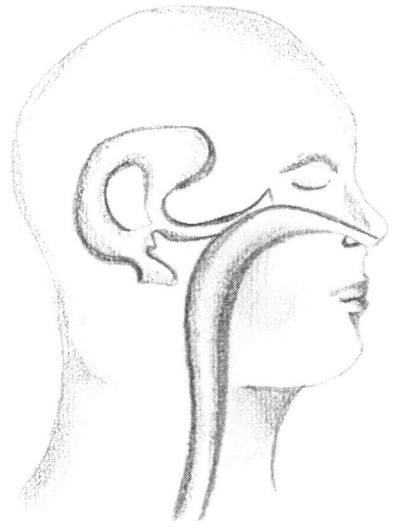

SENSE OF SMELL

The Art of Smell

Clairalience, also known as clairessence meaning clear olfaction is another of the extra sensory functions, and refers to the ability to detect the aromas associated with a person or place without them being physically present and like clairvoyance and clairsentience is closely linked with psychic ability.

It is a skill that can easily go unnoticed yet sometimes an unrelated aroma seems to suddenly appear from nowhere to trigger a powerful memory. All too often we put this down to coincidence but if we allow ourselves to believe, this enables us to pick up on the unique essence of a person or place throughout the passage of time.

Odour molecules present in the air are taken in through the nose, integrated and interpreted and a decision is made as to their origin, nature, safety and desirability. Certain odour molecules also have the ability to affect changes in the body, depending on their composition and strength. This occurs in the following ways:

- Certain odour molecules are capable of being absorbed directly into the blood stream through the capillaries in the lining of the nose

- Through the lungs, as the odour molecules are inhaled and enter the blood stream during gaseous exchange

- The analysis of odour in the limbic centre of the brain activates the associated memory store

The physiology of the body and mind may be altered as a direct result and aromatherapy describes the treatment of the whole body through smell. Amongst the most effective aromas are those from essential oils which form concentrated liquids that are produced in specialist cells of certain parts of plants, for example:

- Petals eg Rose

- Flowering tops eg Lavender

- Whole flowers eg Jasmine

- Leaves eg Eucalyptus

- Twigs eg Tea Tree

- Grasses eg Palmarosa

- Seeds eg Fennel

- Berries eg Juniper

- Fruit peel or rind eg Lemon

- Wood and bark eg Sandalwood

- Roots eg Vetiver

- Resins and gums eg Frankincense

Each essential oil has a unique fragrance, which identifies it, reflects its chemical composition and may be classified as being a top, middle or base note with the potential to initiate physiological response within the body.

Top notes are the most volatile of the essential oils and as such evaporate quickly. They have a sharp aroma, are very stimulating and have a short-term effect (up to 24 hours). Examples include lemon, tea tree and eucalyptus. Used in perfume, top notes are responsible for the initial olfactory impact.

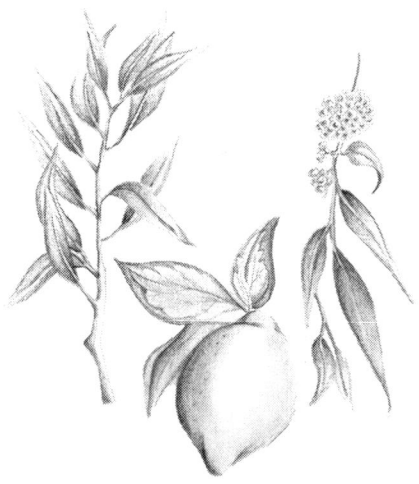

EUCALYPTUS, LEMON, TEA TREE

Middle notes are essential oils that are moderately volatile evaporating at an average rate. Their effects last up to two to three days in the body. Examples include lavender and fennel. Middle notes are also known as heart notes when used in perfumes.

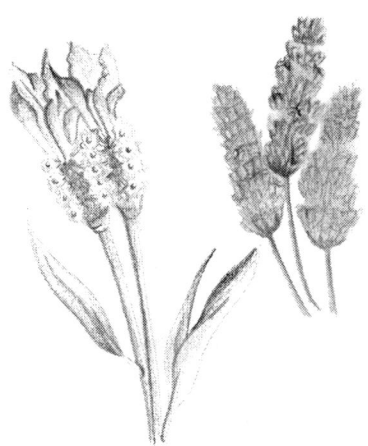

FENNEL AND LAVENDER

Base notes are the slowest essential oils to evaporate. Their effects tend to be more soothing and calming than the other notes and last up to seven days in the body. Examples include rose, frankincense, jasmine and sandalwood. Base notes used in perfumes provide a fragrance with its unique olfactory signature.

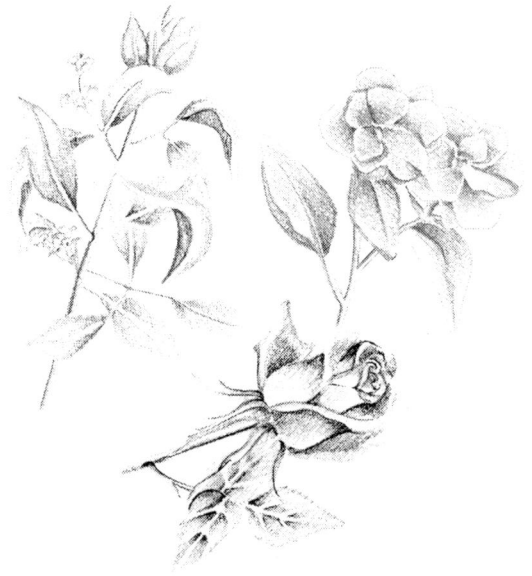

ROSE, JASMINE AND SANDALWOOD

An aromatherapist will combine their study of the body with skilful blending to formulate a synergy of notes to achieve the required therapeutic effect. The resulting blend of essential oils may be simply inhaled and/or added to a base oil to produce a massage medium that can be worked into the skin.

> In perfumery, a nose is someone who uses knowledge, creativity and intuition to produce each new olfactory oracle.

Nose Facts – The Physical Nose

The two passageways in the nose are separated by a thin wall of cartilage known as the septum. These nasal cavities are lined with ciliated mucous membrane, which forms a thin layer of mucus-forming cells that contain tiny hair like structures (cilia) and have a rich blood supply.

Not only does the nose perform the sensory function of smell or olfaction but it also processes the incoming air which is moistened by mucus, filtered by the cilia and warmed by the blood, thus making its journey into the body more comfortable, pleasant and fresh.

Small bones form the bridge and sides of the nose whilst cartilage forms the flexible shape of the front of the nose. The nasalis and procerus muscles cover the nose and contribute to the wrinkling of the skin and the flaring of the nostrils – facial expressions that contribute to non-verbal methods of communication. The nose has strong links with the throat, tongue, eyes, sinuses and ears.

The throat or pharynx consists of the areas at the back of the nose known as the nasopharynx and the back of the mouth known as the oropharnyx and there is a direct link between the two parts. The adenoids are present in the nasopharynx and the tonsils in the oropharynx, which contribute to the immune functions of this area and help to purify the incoming air. The oropharynx leads into the trachea and eventually the lungs.

The nose and tongue share the limbic centre of the brain for the interpretation of smell and taste. Smell occurs whilst breathing in, whilst taste occurs with the outward breath.

The eyes drain excess fluid from the tear-producing lacrimal glands into the nasopharynx which is why crying results in not only streaming eyes but also a runny nose.

The sinuses are air spaces in the facial bones above, below and within the eye sockets that produce mucus, the excess of which also drains into the nasopharynx.

The Eustachian tube connects the middle ear and the back of the nose, enabling pressure to be balanced in the head. This occurs during swallowing and yawning.

As part of the respiratory system the nose is prone to infection from the incoming air, which is easily transferred to these interconnecting areas.

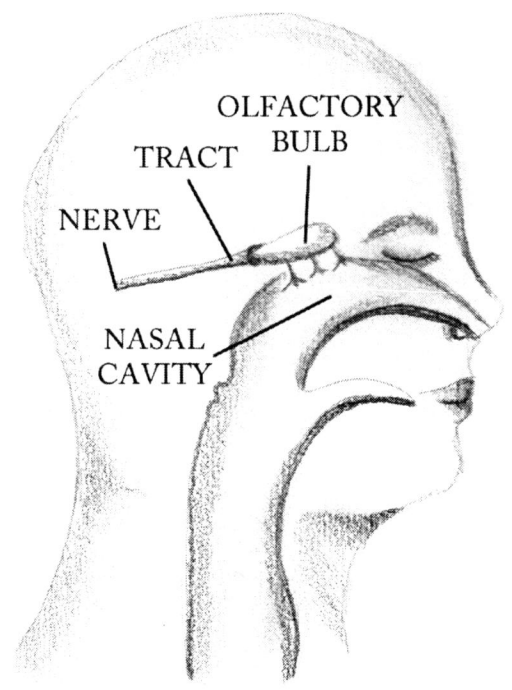

Nose facts – The Emotional Nose

The contraction of the muscles of the nose results in facial expressions which help to communicate a whole set of emotions from nostril-flaring anger to nose-wrinkling distaste.

The sense of smell enables the emotions to be stimulated. Purposeful introduction of aromas may stimulate or soothe the emotions, whilst the sudden appearance of an aroma can initiate strong negative feelings. Aromas that trigger strong personal memories can swiftly stir up a turmoil of emotions and take a person back to a specific time or place in their lives.

> The scent of frangipani flowers conjures up for me in an instant, the memory of climbing the Easy Tree with friends in Singapore so called, because all the neighbourhood children could climb it.

Nose Facts – The Spiritual Nose

The use of aromas to create an atmosphere has long been part of religious and spiritual practices. The word perfume is derived in fact from the Latin *per fumum* – through smoke. The people of ancient worlds found that burning certain natural raw materials gave off beautiful mood-enhancing aromas as well as an accompanying smoke, through which they believed a link between heaven and earth could be created.

The subsequent extraction of essential oils continued to be used as a means to enhance the surrounding air, unblocking stagnant energy in a quest to prepare the mind for spiritual enlightenment. The qualities of the different aromas are said to balance the aura and the chakras, clearing the energy pathways so links to higher levels of consciousness become possible.

Essential oils are reported to hold different properties to achieve differing levels of enlightenment, but personal preference is important. For some the effects of clairalience (ie becoming aware of an unexpected aroma) initiates a desire to use that particular aroma as part of a spiritual journey, whilst meditative practice can help to focus its therapeutic value.

Nose Beauty

The perfect nose should be an eye width at its base, fitting neatly into the middle section of the longitudinal face and within the middle third transversely. The base of the nose in profile should be in a straight line with the base of the forehead at the top and the chin at the bottom. It should be neither too thin nor too upturned and should be strongly built with a gently rounded tip. Nostrils should be pear shaped with clear airways entering the body. Variations between perfect female and male noses should reflect the yin and yang traits associated with soft and hard. The skin covering the nose should be of even texture and colour and free from any evidence of damaged blood vessels, open or blocked pores.

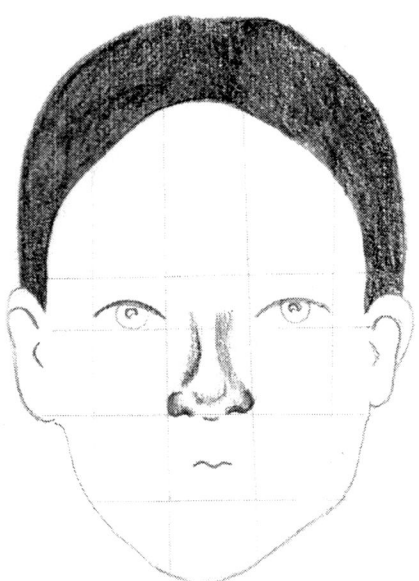

THE PERFECT NOSE

Noses were pierced as long ago as 4,000 years. Like most other forms of piercing the size and quality of the stud or ring was used to display family wealth.

The septum separating the two nostrils in the middle of the nose may be pierced with a ring or bar, and a stud or ring can be inserted on either side of the nose. Nose piercing is a traditional Indian procedure: females commonly pierce the left side of their noses to symbolise fertility and as part of the Ayurvedic paradigm, in the belief that it will ease the pain associated with menstruation and childbirth. Chains may be used to link the nose with similar piercing in the ears to add beauty and glamour to the bearer and reinforce the physiological connections between the two parts of the body.

Nose Power

Not only does olfaction have mood-changing powers, it can also lay claim to the power of synchronisation. Body rhythms between people living and working in close proximity may be affected by the production of human pheromones.

> An example of olfactory power is the synchronisation of menstrual cycles in groups of women who work closely together.

Pheromones are olfactory chemical signals produced in the body and picked up through the process of olfaction. Associated with human identification and development, pheromones provide an olfactory template that can result in human bonding on all levels.

The Language of The Nose

The sense of smell can provide the means for maternal ties as well as sexual attraction, selection and seduction. Pheromones in bodily fluids give out an olfactory signature that bonds a mother and her infant and can also trigger mating behaviour in post pubescent adults.

> The sweat produced by the apocrine glands situated in the groin, underarms and nipples contains pheromones. These glands are activated at puberty initiating an olfactory mating call.

Perfumes are used to simulate and enhance the action of pheromones whilst other fragrances are added to create an atmospheric aroma that appeals to the rest of the senses. Our choice of perfume creates a personal signature on which memories are founded.

Nose Care

As part of the special senses, the nose requires special care.

Water contributes to the production of mucus in the inner lining of the nose helping to moisten the incoming air for added comfort and ease of passageway into the body.

> **Waterworks:** Water intake contributes greatly to the links between the ear, nose and throat. Dehydration can lead to irritation and a loss of clear function. Dairy products are thought to be mucus forming, which if eaten in excess can lead to congestion. Increased water intake helps to cleanse the area and keep mucus free flowing.

Cleanliness and hygiene are vital components of nose care affecting the well-being of the outer skin and inner function:

As part of the T-Zone, the outer skin of the nose contains a greater number of sebum (natural oil) producing glands and is subsequently prone to problems. This skin responds well to beauty routines in terms of:

- Cleansing: to remove any excess sebum and sweat as well as makeup and dust etc. Oil free cleansers and facial washes are great if sebum content and the shine factor are high

- Steaming: gentle heat applied to the central panel of face opens the pores to release congestion. The warmth makes any extraction of the deep plugs of sebum associated with comedones (blackheads) easier

- Exfoliating: chemical exfoliators help to peel away excessive dead skin cells whereas mechanical exfoliators in the form of abrasive creams slough away the offending cells

- Toning: the application of an astringent toning product eg witch hazel will ensure the skin stays oil free as well as helping to refine the pores

- Moisturising: as sebum is a natural protector, moisturising may be kept to a minimum in the case of oily skin. However, the use of a sun protection factor is vital to avoid sun damage

- Masks: clay masks combat the over-secretion of sebum and may be mixed as needed. Kaolin mixed with witch hazel gives an effective drawing action that purifies, tightens and tones

Inner function responds well to remedial practices in terms of:

- Cleansing: due to the moistening and filtering action of the nose the potential for nasal congestion and infection is high. Splashing water into the nostrils followed by blowing the nose helps to clear and cleanse. Breathing is easier and if done last thing at night, sleep may be enhanced

- Inhalations: the combined action of steam together with the therapeutic properties of certain essential oils eg eucalyptus have the effect of clearing the airways helping to decongest, improve breathing and purify and strengthen the airways

- Ear candling: the treatment, also known as thermal auricular therapy, has a therapeutic effect on all of the areas linked to the ears including the nose through its action of clearing the Eustachian tube. This aids inflammation, irritation and congestion in the nose as well as being ultra-relaxing which in turn aids breathing

Olfactory defects should be taken seriously and medical advice sought. **Anosmia** refers to the loss of the sense of smell and may be a temporary or permanent condition. Whilst not as crucial to the quality of life as the loss of some of the other sensory functions like sight or hearing, this has been linked with depression and lack of libido. Specific Anosmia describes being unable to identify a specific aroma.

> Hyposmia refers to a decreasing ability to smell and often occurs as a result of the ageing process.
>
> Hyperosmia refers to a heightened sense of smell and can accompany some forms of illness.

Like all the sensory organs, the nose adapts to constant exposure to an aroma and after a while stops reacting to it.

> The wearer of a perfume stops smelling it after a while, while others with whom they come into contact remain aware of the aroma unless they spend a long time together.

Exposing the olfactory system to a variety of different aromas can lift and open the mind and may be used to aid relaxation, prepare for meditation, stimulate concentration, encourage focus, enhance a therapeutic treatment, inspire creativity, rekindle romance and fuel desire.

> When choosing different essential oils for their aroma and therapeutic value, it is important that the person making the choice likes the fragrance. As the internal environment of the body changes through its natural cycles eg sleep/wake, menstrual etc different aromas evoke different responses. As a general rule of thumb, if the smell of an aroma is offensive in any way it should be avoided until such time, if ever, that it becomes desirable.

In yogic practices it is believed that the nose is a vehicle by which to evolve towards a higher level of consciousness and spirituality. Cleansing and purification practices may be used to ensure that the journey runs smoothly.

> **Neti:** Neti refers to a cleansing and purification process of the nose. There are two types of neti:
>
> Sutri neti - a piece of waxed cord is dipped in lukewarm, salty water and inserted into one nostril. As the tip of the cord emerges at the back of the mouth, it can be slowly pulled out before repeating the process on the other side.
>
> Jala neti - using a small pot with a suitable spout, lukewarm, salty water is poured into one nostril and with the head tipped, emerges from the other. This should be repeated on both sides after which any excess may be blown out. In the case of a blocked nostril the water will emerge from the mouth and may be spat out.
>
> Both procedures are not for the faint hearted but once mastered, may be used daily.

Scent Scene

The word *aroma* is the Latin word for seasoning and spice.

All manner of fragrant aromas were used by early man to help make sense of their existence in the world and to reinforce their growing religious beliefs. As human bodily scents ensured the attraction of the sexes, it was believed that other naturally occurring aromas ensured the attraction of the gods paving the way for a better here and now as well as a more fruitful after life. Raw materials were often burnt with the resulting smoke offering a passageway for thoughts and prayers to reach the heavens whilst the fragrant aromas could be used to soothe or stimulate human and heavenly senses. Thus incense became associated with immortality and perfume accompanied the death rituals of the past and present alike.

Frankincense and myrrh share a strong religious history.

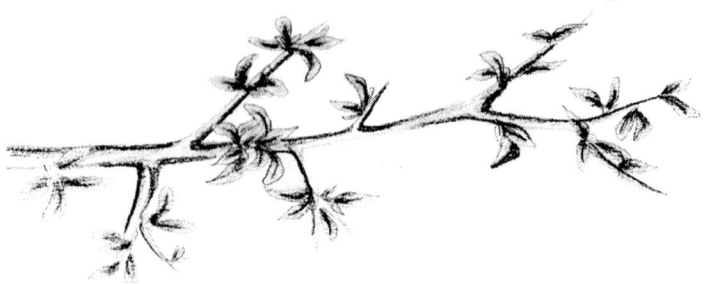

MYRRH

In addition to the burning of some fragrant raw materials the essential oils of others were extracted in a variety of ways with their methods becoming more sophisticated, scientific and profitable as the ancient and modern worlds developed.

Enfleurage describes an ancient and thus nowadays lesser-used, highly expensive method of extraction reserved for the very finest fragrances.

Fresh flowers are laid onto plates containing highly refined and odourless fat.

Over a period of time further flowers are added whilst others are discarded until the fat has absorbed the required amount of essential oils.

The saturated fat is known as **pomade,** which is washed in alcohol and the residue fat discarded before being heated to release the essential oil.

Maceration describes a method of extraction similar to enfleurage whereby the raw materials are placed in hot fat, which penetrates the plants cells absorbing the essential oil, which is then released in a similar way to the latter stages of enfleurage.

Steam distillation is a more common method of extraction, resulting in an essential oil and fragrant water eg rose oil and rose water.

Steam passes through raw material such as the rose petals.

The heat releases the natural oil, which then becomes suspended in the steam.

The oil-filled steam is captured in a vessel where the steam turns back into water and the oil and water separate. The oil contains the powerful inherent fragrance of the raw material hence the term 'essential oil' whilst the water contains only faint traces.

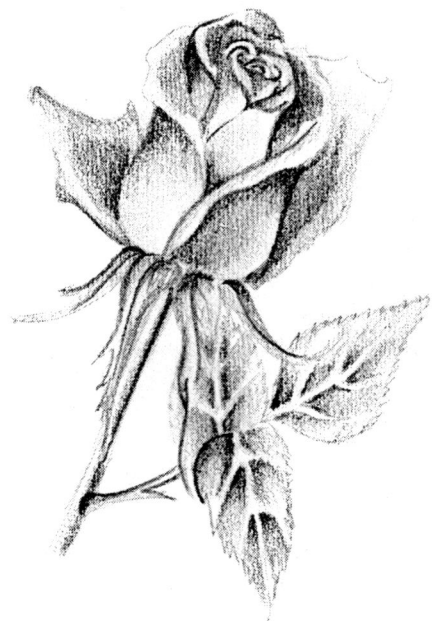

Expression describes a common method of extracting essential oils from citrus fruits, updated from traditional methods.

The peel/zest is removed and placed within mechanical crushers that press out the oil and juice.

The watery juice is separated leaving behind the zesty essential oil.

> Before the use of machines, the fruit peel was grated or squeezed by hand into a sponge and the essential oils drained off and stored. Many workers experienced severe allergic reactions.

Solvent extraction results in an essential oil that bears the true-to-life fragrance of its raw material known as an **absolute**.

A solvent is passed through the raw material absorbing its fragrant oil before being mixed with it.

Once spent the raw material is discarded. The resulting product is a waxy paste known as a **concrete** if from a fresh raw material such as flowers or a **resinoid** if from a dry raw material such as wood.

Further processing removes the waxes leaving a mixture of essential oil and alcohol.

This mixture is sensitively heated to evaporate the alcohol without damaging the essential oil.

Throughout history, the resulting fragrant essential oils together with animal products and the introduction in later years of synthetic additions have all been used to create unique aromatic blends which are formulated into perfumes of varying strengths and/or added to a whole host of health and beauty products for their therapeutic value as well as for their unique aromas including unguents and pomades, and the ointments, mouthwashes, creams and lotions, shampoos and conditioners of today.

Animal products that have been used in perfumes include:

- Civet: a paste from the civet cat with a distinct faecal odour was commonly used in gentlemen's fragrances in 18th century

- Musk: obtained from a gland situated between the back/rectal areas of the male Musk deer providing a deep sensual aroma

- Castoreum: the dried secretion of castor sacs of mature North American and European beavers, which gives off a leathery aroma. Used in some classic perfumes such as Guerlain's Shalimar

- Ambergris: a solid, waxy substance produced in the digestive systems of sperm whales. Ambergris is regurgitated by the whales and is harvested floating on the sea's surface or lying on coastal sands.

Animal products are understandably expensive and their use controversial today. Synthetic replicas are thus common.

The social use of perfume has changed over the years.

The bodies of ancient royalty were embalmed with perfumes and a variety of artefacts have been found that were once used to give off beautiful and meaningful aromas to accompany funeral rites and rituals and adorn their tombs, ensuring that these most revered of humans would enjoy equal status in their afterlife.

Just as prayers were believed to travel to the heavens via fragrant smoke so too could a person's spirit and the frequent use of such fragrances helped to keep the spirit alive and well. As a result, perfumes became prized for their earthly and ethereal value and continued to create a phenomenon that the development of the ancient and modern worlds has never lost sight of.

Apart from being used for religious practices, perfumes were also used to ward off evil spirits and keep disease at bay.

> The phrase 'to keep at bay' comes from the use of bay leaves thought to ward off the plague.

Perfumes were used to cover up the unpleasant smells of bodies, living quarters and even animals as well create the seductive aromas on offer today.

> Floors would be covered with flowers and herbs, pillows filled with petals and scented oils rubbed into the skins of animals as well as people. The leather that was used in the making of fine gloves was frequently softened and fragranced by essential oils. Pomades would be worn by men and women and frequently wafted at approaching bad smells. Rosary beads could be scented to make for more pleasant religious devotion and ladies' fans sprayed with perfume emitting beautiful fragrances with every flick of the wrist. Strong smelling salts were used to reawaken the weak from a dose of the vapours and foul odorous wounds were treated with healing unguents and compresses doused in essential oils to disguise the smell of decay.

The Romans - famous for their health and hygiene and the pleasure they took in looking after the body - first brought perfumes to Britain. As travel opened up the world, the trade in perfumes grew, with many essential oils commanding a value equal to that of the most precious of jewels.

However, perfume, like health, beauty and makeup products, has enjoyed a varied and colourful history, with fragrance fashions changing with each new generation.

As well as being wafted and waved, doused and dabbed, they have also been drunk as elixirs of youth.

As such, perfumes have taken centre stage, attracting cult status yet also sharing strong associations with prostitution and low morals.

As health and hygiene eventually took on greater meaning in the modern world, so too did the manufacture of products, with methods of extraction becoming easier and less costly. Instead of covering up the bad aromas that accompanied poor hygiene and failing health, perfumes were used to enhance the cleansing and moisturising properties of mass-produced products. The once great unwashed gradually became the great washed, cleaned and fragrant.

Natural versus Synthetic

With world travel came trade in raw materials, advances in methods of extraction, and the introduction of synthetic materials.

The raw materials of perfume are either natural or synthetic:

- **Natural aroma products** are essential oils retrieved directly from nature, have always been available and trial and error have formed their therapeutic and fragrant development. Essential oils have a long tradition of use and are associated with time-consuming, creative and costly cottage industries.

- **Synthetic aroma products** on the other hand are manmade. First used commercially in 1889 they have gone on to shape the perfume industry with their complexity, flexibility and ability to be more cost effectively mass-produced. And whilst the term synthetic conjures up a sterile, clinical and artificially manufactured image that is viewed by some as being negative, synthetics may be used in some cases to purify, refine, etherealise and elevate the naturals.

The myriad fragrances available from the mix of natural and synthetic aromas fall into the following categories

- **Perfume:** the finest and costliest form of fragrance, with the highest percentage of aroma products (between 20-40%) within pure alcohol. Perfumes have a greater concentration of base notes, which makes them last longer than all other forms of fragrance.

- **Eau de Parfum (EDP):** fewer aroma products within 90% proof alcohol. A smaller concentration of base note is used so its staying power is less than that of perfume.

- **Eau de Toilette (EDT):** contains substantially fewer aroma products to alcohol with a smaller concentration of base notes, so its aroma is shorter lived.

- **Eau de Cologne:** developed in Cologne in the 1730s. Top note aroma products dominate, so a fresh and uplifting, albeit short-term fragrance.
- **Eau Fraiche:** between eau de toilette and eau de cologne, with the freshness of cologne and the increased longevity of toilette.

With so many fragrant products on the market, it might be said that science has all but taken over from the art of perfume making, which in turn has led to the perfume-for-profit phenomena. This is a result of the science of mass production and creative media hype which work together to produce and sell quick-fix perfumes (usually celebrity endorsed) to suit lifestyles, meet the high demands of fashion and accompany changing cultural and social mood.

Underlying all this however, is the art of creation and innovation that favours quality over cost.

Can Real Beauty Be Found in a Spritz or Spray?

Perfumes are non-judgmental, always willing to not only share with us their beauty but also their profound effect. With little regard to age they imprint on the mind a unique message that transcends time and space.

Often referred to as 'glamour in a bottle' perfume brands make many claims that we are all too happy to buy into. Their very names promise us delivery of the essence of beauty. As we take from nature the most beautiful of its aromas in a quest to emulate its qualities in order to enhance those of our own our choices reflect our experiences and influences, our memories and feelings and our aspirations and dreams. Coco Chanel believed that women should wear perfume wherever they hoped to be kissed. This works well on those areas where the blood is closest to the surface and warms the perfume to release its fragrant beauty ie wrist, elbow, back of the knee.

> When applying perfume to the wrists, they should not be rubbed together as this crushes and damages the aroma molecules. Layering of perfumed products works to keep the wearer in a cloud of scent as each one releases its aromas. Many fragrance houses will have shower/bath, moisturising and perfume products for such pampering effects.
>
> Perfumes are volatile and delicate. They benefit from being stored away from direct sunlight to maintain their essence.

We all of us have a perfume diary – a history of unique fragrances that have helped to shape our lives.

My own starts with my German mother's favourite, 4711, and my father's Christmas splashes of Old Spice that filled my childhood.

> ### Olfactory Origins
>
> 4711: named after the residence of a Cologne merchant Wilhelm Mülhens 4711 is his version of the original Eau de Cologne which was first produced in 1709 by Italian perfumer Giovanni Maria Farina.

> Old Spice: made its first appearance in America in 1937 as a woman's fragrance called Early American Old Spice. This was followed in 1938 by Old Spice for men which went on to become the largest-selling mass produced men's aftershave. Its masculine nautical trademark enjoyed universal appeal. In 2008 Old Spice was updated and repackaged, an example of a new fragrance bearing little or no resemblance to the original classic, much to the dismay of its fans.

Faberge's Brut accompanied me into puberty. Costing all of 50p for a miniature bottle in a box, we girls would buy it for our dads and splash it all over (Henry Cooper style) before a night out roller skating, mindless of the mixed messages we must have been wafting in our wake!

> Faberge's Brut was launched in 1964 as 'the essence of man' and has a long history of sporting endorsements with the likes of Mohammed Ali in America and Henry Cooper in the UK. Elvis is even reported to have worn it.

Next came Revlon's iconic Charlie, which I shared with my mother as liberated and united females. Introduced in 1973, Charlie was affordable, ultra modern and captured the mood of the moment.

> Created for Revlon by the perfumer Francis Camail, Charlie was an aromatic blend of many elements that provided an almost universal appeal. Charlie went on to become a perfume sensation that defined the changing attitudes of and towards women.

My move to London and the start of my career in beauty gave me unrivalled access to all that was expensive, exclusive and extravagant opening my olfactory eyes (if not my purse) to the aspirations and opulence of Jean Patou's Joy. As I walked through Harrods perfumery on my way to work I enjoyed its joyousness from afar.

> Heralded as the costliest perfume in the world, Joy was made from the most precious raw materials and sold in a beautifully-crafted Baccarat bottle. It has been given the accolade of being the scent of the 20th century .

During my young, free and single years I had a yearning for Estée Lauder's Youth Dew, flirted with Fidji by Guy Laroche, dabbled with the Dior set and courted Chanel before having a full on love affair with Yves Saint Laurent's Rive Gauche.

> Realising that women felt guilty buying perfume for themselves, Estée Lauder created Youth Dew as a concentrated bath oil, which applied to the skin after bathing became a cheaper alternative to the expensive bottles of perfumes but with much of its lasting fragrance.
>
> Guy Laroche conjured up a seductive image with the introduction of Fidji in 1966 with the words 'A woman is an island, Fidji is her perfume' and precipitated the start of a universal move to tell a story when advertising a fragrance.
>
> From the introduction of the New Look Dior reached even higher levels of luxury with each new venture from Miss Dior (1947) , Diorama (1949), Diorissimo (1956), Diorella (1972) and Dioressence (1979) legendary scents some of which have stood the test of time.
>
> Coco Chanel's launch of Chanel No 5 in the 1920s was instrumental in creating the now unbreakable links that bind fashion, fragrance and beauty enabling couture scents to become the ultimate accessory.
>
> Taking over from Dior, Yves Saint Laurent went on to achieve great perfume success to match that of his couture with the launch of the highly acclaimed Rive Gauche.

My earliest memories of my husband are cloaked in Dior's Eau Savage, marketed as the ultimate expression of masculinity, whilst the lasting memory of my late father will always be found in Estée Lauder's Aramis.

> Eau Savage was launched nine years after Dior's death and was the first fragrance to use a natural isolate (one small element of a natural aroma product) known as dihydrojasmonate, which has a fresh citrus-like aroma that is long lasting. Nowadays dihydrojasmonate is widely used.
>
> Launched in 1964 Aramis paved the way for men's grooming, introducing male beauty products for face, hair and body. Heralding himself as a New Man my father revelled in his iconic soap on a rope and the free umbrella that accompanied the gift-with-purchase campaign each year.

My engagement was steeped in Paco Rabanne, whilst my wedding day was veiled in Eau de Givenchy. Both gifts from my husband to be, Eau de Givenchy continued to mist the early days of our marriage and even fragranced the hospital air (along with blood, sweat and tears) whilst I gave birth to our daughter.

Calvin Klein's Escape and Eternity brought perfume unity to the next stages of our marriage with his and hers homogeneity, and the powerful strength of Giorgio Beverly Hills featured as an olfactory must-have whilst I developed my business.

> Paco Rabanne scents were of an unconventional nature to match his couture.

> Calvin Klein started his perfume journey with Obsession followed by Eternity and Escape but it was CK1 that made the most impact with a unisex scent in sync with the trends of the decade.
>
> Women who wore Giorgio left behind a trail of scent like none other and it soon became synonymous with the Dallas and Dynasty in-your-face style of beauty along with the power dressing of the era.

Subtlety replaced strength and peace took over power for a while with Clarins' Eau Dynamisante and Clinique's Happy. However, the lure of the designer soon had me matching my perfumes, handbags and jewellery with the likes of Issey Miyake, Marc Jacobs and Chopard with my mother and my daughter sharing in our joint quest for perfume supremacy.

> Skincare and Makeup houses like Clarins and Clinique developed treatment fragrances with a more holistic approach to their fragrance. Light and airy, their scent was designed to reflect health and wellbeing.
>
> Issey Miyake and Marc Jacobs met the needs of the era with designer label scents to reflect the simplicity and style or their designer label couture.
>
> Chopard is famous for its exceptionally fine watches, jewellery and complimentary fragrances. Founded in 1860, it wasn't until 1963 that they started to make jewellery and the fragrances that reflect their opulent beauty.

With hot flushes and dipping blood pressure came a need to keep it real and a penchant for Penhaligon developed. Their Lily and Spice transports me straight back to my childhood tree climbing days in Singapore. Bluebell conjures up the freshness of spring, whilst Elizabethan Rose and Violetta evoke feminine, nostalgic and nurturing tendencies.

> The English perfume house of Penhaligon was founded in the late 1800s by William Henry Penhaligon who went on to become the court barber and perfumer to Queen Victoria. He opened a shop in London's Jermyn Street, which was destroyed during the war in 1941. Penhaligon was newly opened in 1975 by fashion designer Sheila Pickles with the help of the film director Franco Zeffirelli. Many of the old recipes were resurrected and exciting new fragrances launched, all reminiscent of a bygone era.

Not only do we each possess our unique perfume diary, most men as well as women nowadays also own an eclectic perfume wardrobe. Whether our choices celebrate perfume for profit, perfume for potential or even a healthy mix of the two, there is no denying that the quest for beauty lies behind each purchase.

Whilst it may be a conscious choice of the ego (I need to be like the celebrity whose name endorses the perfume) or the subconscious choice of the Id (being intuitively drawn to the essence of a fragrance) our mind is made up only when a sense of beauty is being experienced.

CHAPTER FIVE

Taste

Smell and taste are in fact but a single composite

sense, whose laboratory is the mouth and

its chimney the nose

Anthelme Brillat-Savarin

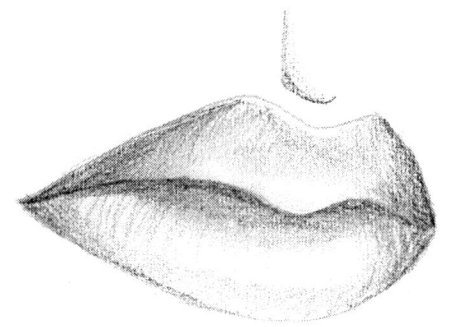

The Science of Taste

The sensory function associated with taste is known as **gustation** and takes place not only on the tongue but also along the soft palate and the surfaces of the **pharynx** and **epiglottis**. Taste buds or receptor cells receive the various different flavours, which are then carried to the **limbic centre** of the brain via the seventh and ninth **cranial nerves** also known as the **facial** and **glossopharyngeal** nerves whereby the various qualities of taste are recognised and identified.

Because of the close links in the brain between the areas responsible for analysing taste and smell it is often difficult to differentiate between smell and taste. As one of the subtler yet highly sensitive sensory functions, gustation along with olfaction contributes to the more intimate judgments of beauty.

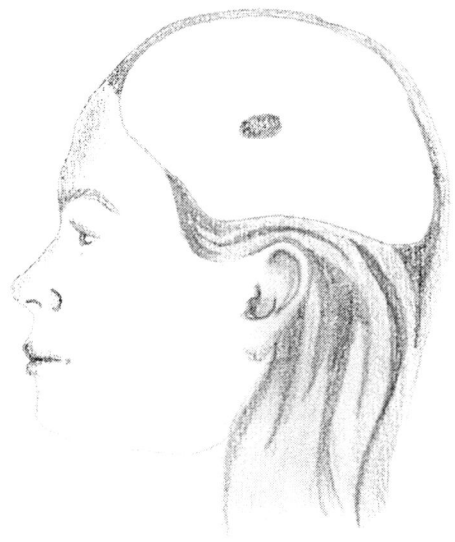

SENSE OF TASTE

In the west, experts have identified four main taste sensations including sweet, sour, salty and bitter flavors, and two more have been identified by the eastern cultures.

In Japanese the term *umami* describes good flavour and may be interpreted as being associated with a savoury taste. *Piquance* is considered to be the sixth taste sensation and describes that which is hot and spicy.

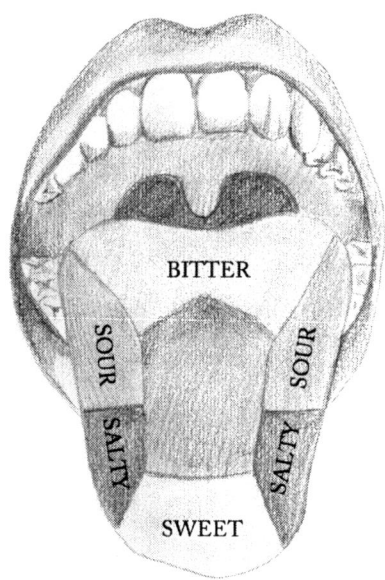

The Art of Taste

Clairgustance, clear taste, refers to a taste sensation without the tongue or indeed any part of the mouth coming into physical contact with taste releasing particles. This may occur in conjunction with clairalience or alone and is thought to signify the non-physical presence of that which may be associated with taste and smell.

The Tongue Tells The Truth, The Whole Truth and Nothing But The Truth

The tongue is another area of the physique that offers the promise of analysis of the rest of the body forming a single part that has the ability to reflect more than just itself. Tongue analysis takes its origins from the eastern cultures of Ayurveda and Chinese Traditional Medicine and is known as *yetsu shin* in Japanese.

Whilst the location of the organs in the map of the body on the tongue is subject to differing views there is a universal belief in the fact that the well-being of the body is reflected in the condition of the tongue. Analysis involves the checking of the tongue's shape, texture, movement, coating and moisture levels, which is carried out by some as a daily means of self-diagnosis as part of personal care and hygiene as well as a reliable method for medical practitioners to form or confirm a more formal diagnosis.

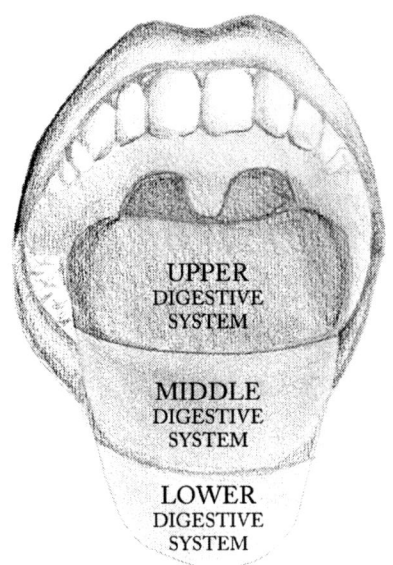

Tongue Facts – The Physical Tongue

The tongue is a muscular structure of eight individual muscles. Of these, four are responsible for controlling the position of the tongue and are attached to the **hyoid** and **mandible** bones of the throat and jaw whilst the remaining four change the shape of the tongue during mastication (chewing) and speech.

The tongue is protected by the mouth and lips, which are formed from a circular muscle called the **orbicularis oris**. This muscle is similar to that which encircles the eyes and is responsible for puckering the lips and contributing to the fine lines that develop around the mouth with age.

The lips contain a rich blood and nerve supply which gives them their distinct colour as well as enabling them to detect the temperature of food and fluid before it enters the mouth.

The **temporalis, buccinator** and **masseter** muscles of the temple and cheek along with the teeth contribute to the mechanical action of chewing, whilst three sets of salivary glands commence chemical digestion in the mouth. The tongue contributes to the process of digestion by rolling the food around the mouth before passing it to the throat for swallowing. It is also responsible for helping to shape the air exiting the body through the mouth during speech in a process known as **phonetic articulation**.

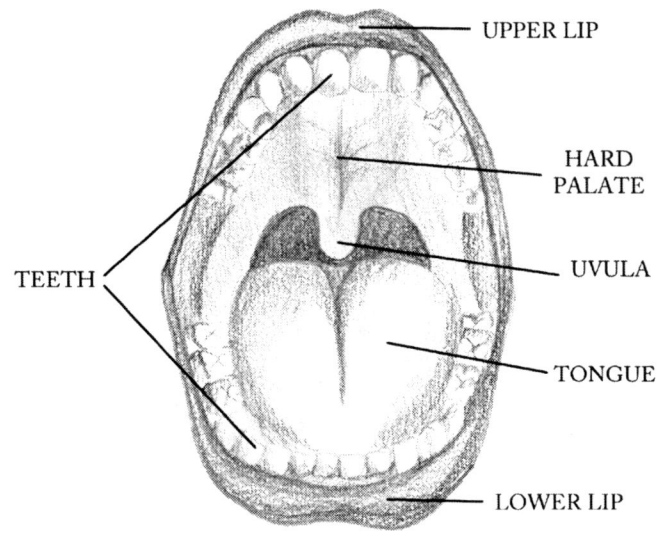

Tongue Facts – The Emotional Tongue

The flexibility of the tongue helps to shape the air exiting the body through the mouth. This is linked to the expressions of thought and emotions through formation of the spoken word. A freely moveable tongue is associated with a freedom of speech and loose talk whilst a less flexible tongue may be linked to a more clipped manner of speech and the inability to express emotions without restraint.

A person may be tight lipped, with the tongue seemingly imprisoned within the mouth rendering them incapable or unwilling to express their true feelings. Being tongue-tied refers to confused speech and a lack of coherent thought which may accompany a bewildered or fearful mind.

We may at times be forced or encouraged to bite or hold our tongue to prevent emotion from escaping (a slip of the tongue) that may either prove too revealing and/or be hurtful to the recipient.

Tongue Facts – The Spiritual Tongue

In addition to spiritual connections with clairgustance the spiritual tongue is also believed by some to explain the use of speech that has been activated by a force other than the person themselves and is often referred to as talking in tongues. Talking in tongues or glossolalia entails the verbal use of consonants and vowels in a limited number of syllables with varying pitch, volume and speed, which may accompany a religious and/or spiritual experience. Another form of talking in tongues refers to the speaking or understanding of an unknown language and is known as xenoglossy. These practices are commonly associated with fanaticism, treated with scepticism and as such viewed with fear and trepidation. However, as with all things spiritual there is much to discover and lots yet to learn.

Tongue Beauty

The perfect tongue should be of a good size, smooth and clear in texture and even in shape. It should be a rich, deep red and agile in movement. A perfect tongue should be comfortably housed within the perfect mouth, which should be of a well-proportioned shape with the lower lip slightly fuller than the upper. The corners of the mouth should be slightly upturned. The gums should not be visible upon smiling and there should be no more than two thirds of the length of the upper front incisor teeth on show.

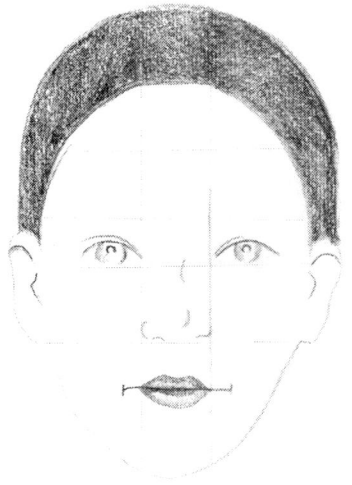

THE PERFECT MOUTH

The tongue and indeed the lips, teeth and mouth in general have a long history associated with beautification. Lip painting, tongue piercing, application of tooth gems and mouth stretching are procedures that have been used by many worldwide cultures and traditions not only as signs of beauty and attraction but also as a means to ward off evil, honour the gods, as rites of passage, to demonstrate social and economic status and in some cases such as with the punk passion for piercing, associated with acts of rebellion.

Lip stretching is one of the lesser commonly accepted methods of beautification and involves increasingly sized discs being inserted into a pierced hole in either or both of the lips of men and women. Social and economic status rather than physical aesthetics was judged by the size of the final disc with the larger discs inevitably holding the greatest attraction and commanding the greatest attention!

Tongue Power

The tongue is like a sharp knife...
kills without drawing blood

Buddha

The tongue is a powerful combination of muscles with the strength to contribute to mechanical digestion and speech articulation as well as take part in the creation of facial expressions and non-verbal body language. The poking out of the tongue forms one of the primary methods of communication in a baby continuing into childhood as a means of rude expression, which may be viewed as an obscenity in its use by adults. However it is viewed, it carries with it the power to produce and affect extreme emotional responses.

'Tongue in cheek' was formerly a physical sign of the powerful emotions associated with contempt that over time has become an expression of a comical or jocular nature ie not to be taken at face value.

> **Tongue Power:** Some people have the power to roll their tongue whilst others are unable to do so no matter how hard they try. It is thought that the ability to roll the tongue in this way is a genetic function produced by a gene that is not dominant or in some cases not even present.

The Language of The Tongue

Phonetic articulation enables a person to learn the complexities associated with language. A person learns their mother tongue by imitating the shapes formed by the muscles of the tongue, mouth and jaw of their carers (usually their mother hence the term). Speed, tone and intonation are added and finally phrases and sentences complete the function of verbal communication whilst knowledge, understanding and awareness contribute to its art. Combining these factors with the subtleties associated with body language enables a person's deeper identity to be acknowledged and pays tribute to the beauty that lies within.

> Licking the lips is non-verbal sign that communicates pleasure and excess and has strong associations with greed and gluttony as well as the simple enjoyment of anticipation and taste of food.
>
> Lip service is an expression used to convey insincere approval or support.

Tongue Care

As part of the special senses, the tongue and the surrounding lips and mouth together with its structures require special care to maintain their function and beauty.

Water intake contributes to the formation of saliva in the mouth, which is necessary not only to keep the area well hydrated but also to aid the process of mechanical and chemical digestion.

> **Waterworks:** Wet saliva mixes with the food to form a swallowable ball known as a bolus, whilst the various enzymes present in saliva start to break down the nutrients ready for absorption.

Rest is a vital component for the wellbeing of the tongue, an area of the body capable of demonstrating the symptoms associated with high stress levels. The position of the tongue pushed firmly against the front teeth, a tightness of the jaw together with the grinding of teeth are all signs of stress which are too often ignored.

> The relaxed jaw should be loose so that the lips are slightly parted. The teeth should not be touching and the tongue should rest comfortably in the centre of the mouth.

Jaw ache refers to the tension that occurs when the mouth is held tight, the lips are pursed, the tongue stiff and the top set of teeth pressed firmly against the bottom set. The muscles of the tongue and surrounding area become strained and overworked resulting in pain and discomfort. Continuous strain will result in the grinding away of tooth enamel. Tongue function may also be affected when tight and strained facial muscles impede nerve responses.

> Mouth exercises and self-massage are an ideal way to keep tension at bay
>
> - Opening the mouth as wide as possible whilst poking out the tongue to stretch the muscles
> - Moving the tongue up and down, to the left and right and around in circles with an open mouth together with exaggerated mouthing of the vowel sounds will strengthen and tone the muscles
> - Circular massage movements to the centre of the cheek relieves tightness in the masseter muscles responsible for jaw movements

Whilst the tongue is able to reflect changes in the body, the mouth is a prime area for infection and decay if uncared for. Regular dental checkups involve the inspection of the mouth as a whole including the tongue, gums, salivary glands and nearby lymph nodes that contribute to the immunity of the body and reflect its general health.

> Gum disease is the main cause of tooth loss and comes in two forms:
>
> - Gingivitis: inflammation resulting in bleeding and sore gums which can if left untreated result in periodontal disease, affecting the underlying jaw bones that hold the sockets for the teeth.
> - Periodontal disease: affecting the underlying jaw bones that hold the sockets for the teeth.

Any changes in the tongue's ability to detect taste should be taken seriously and medical advice sought. These changes may be temporary (the inability to taste when suffering with a bad cold or flu or through vitamin and mineral deficiency eg vitamin B3 and zinc) and may accompany feelings of anxiety as well as being symptoms of more serious underlying conditions.

> Ageusia refers to the loss of taste sensation
>
> Hypogeusia describes a partial loss of taste sensation
>
> Dysgeusia refers to changing taste sensations

Whilst ageing may bring with it a gradual reduction of the sensory functions, premature ageing results in the telltale signs of dropped contours and associated lines and wrinkles around the mouth.

> Smoking is the single most serious contributor to premature ageing of the tongue and mouth. Not only does it hinder the sensory function of taste, it also encourages the build up of bacterial plaque, contributing to gum disease, and causes the early appearance of the lines and wrinkles that threaten to spoil a firm lip line.

The application of products to enhance the natural beauty of the lips may also be applied to create the illusion of perfection by correcting and balancing shape and structure.

> ## Lip Makeup
>
> - To correct lip shape and size:
> - Apply foundation over the entire lip
> - Draw a correcting lip line with a lip pencil within the natural lip line to create a smaller image or outside of the natural lip line to create a larger image
> - Fill in the lips with a corresponding lipstick or gloss, remembering that light colours will create a larger illusion and dark colours the opposite
> - Lip-gloss will add sparkle and shine, drawing further attention to the lips.

The tongue and skin of the lips benefits from a routine of daily cleansing and protecting with the use of remedial treatments like balms, exfoliators and masks as regular and much needed beauty boosts.

Cleansing

Tongue scraping can help to clear away excessive residue that may be coating the surface of tongue.

Gentle cleansers may be used to dissolve stubborn lipstick without fear of damage. A suitable cleansing product should be applied with gentle massage movements and removed with the aid of a damp cotton wool pad.

Protecting

Lip balms and creams shield the fine skin of the lips and may be applied instead of, under or over lipstick. Some lip products contain sun protection factors helping to prevent sun damage if used correctly.

Exfoliation

Gentle abrasive products in the form of exfoliators used for the face may be safely and effectively used on the lips to slough away the build up of dead skin cells leaving the underlying skin smooth and more absorbent.

Masks

Regular application of a nourishing mask supplements the moisture levels of the skin of the lips and surrounding area. This has the effect of boosting moisture content and keeping cells plumped.

The emotional tongue benefits from emotional balance and support. Having the opportunity to let off steam enables the release of pent up emotions that may otherwise manifest themselves in anger and frustration and be expressed as verbal abuse.

Laughter therapy is a means to not only exercise the muscles of the mouth and tongue but also to encourage a positive release of emotions, reducing stress levels to be replaced with a higher feel good factor. It is reported that children laugh on average 300-400 times a day but adults only around 15 times a day.

Meditative practices and the use of visualisations and affirmations may result in a greater sense of awareness of the spiritual tongue and may lead to more ready acceptance of inherent yet underdeveloped skills.

> Visualisation – imaging with the mind's eye a tongue that is flexible and free sends a strong message to the mouth, which in time begins to act upon the vision.
>
> Affirmation – reinforcing the vision of a freely moveable tongue with a positive thought relating to the freedom of speech encourages this as a reality.

Breathe, Drink, Eat, Love and Live

A human organism is comprised of millions of individual cells that each rely on nutrients for their continued form, function, well-being and ultimate survival.

Cells form the building blocks from which a human being develops, grows and matures. The structure and function of cells reflect that of a fully-formed person. Each contains a set of **organelles** or little organs capable of maintaining life ie through the processes of respiration, metabolism, excretion, movement, sensation and reproduction.

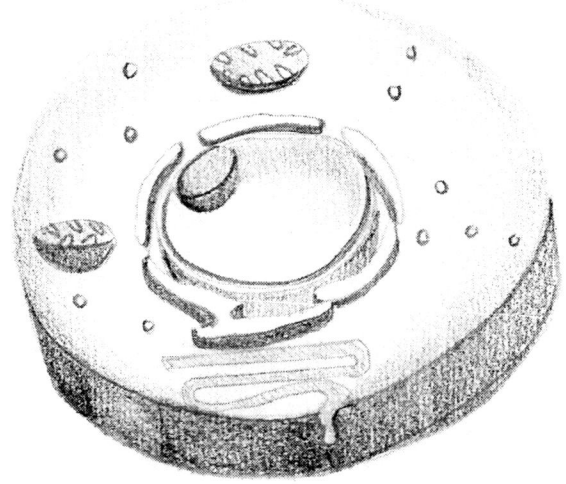

BUILDING BLOCK – A CELL

Once formed, like-minded cells group together to form tissue. There are four types of tissue including:

- Epithelial tissue: groups of cells that form the linings of organs and the coverings of the body. Protective in its nature, epithelial tissue may be multi layered eg the surface of the skin, the hair and the nails

- Connective tissue: groups of cells that link the body including the blood, bones, cartilage, tendons and ligaments etc.

- Muscular tissue: groups of cells capable of the involuntary movement associated with organs of the body as well as the voluntary movement of the skeletal muscles.

- Nervous tissue: groups of cells providing the body with the ability to sense and respond via the interaction of sensory and motor nerves with the brain and spinal cord.

Glands and organs are formed from a combination of these tissue types as further groupings produce multi functional body systems, which ultimately lead to the development of a fully functioning human organism.

> **Cell Power:** It is worth noting that a single cell can do anything a fully-formed human being can do, on a miniature scale.

Individual cells have a limited programmed life span which undergoes a constant process of renewal known as **mitosis** or simple cell division, dependent on nutritional input.

Nutrients may be described as being something with the power to nourish and whilst food is the most obvious example, oxygen, water, love and light all play a vital role.

Oxygen - often described as our life force - is the fundamental nutrient without which life cannot be sustained for more than a few moments.

> Air contains a mixture of gases that form the atmosphere in which we live. It is composed of nitrogen, oxygen and other gases including carbon dioxide, with varying amounts of moisture, pollution and dust etc.

The Science of Breathing

Breathing in and out is a continuous cycle that binds us to the surrounding environment. The carbon dioxide we breathe out is used by plant life during photosynthesis to produce the oxygen we breathe in. This interaction is known as **external respiration,** and has two distinct phases:

Inspiration – Breathing In

- The diaphragm contracts pushing the abdominal cavity down.

- The intercostal muscles that entwine the ribs contract to pull the ribs up and out.

- The thoracic cavity enlarges and the pressure within the lungs decreases.

- Air rushes into the body with increased pressure expanding the lungs.

> Household dust is comprised of a large percentage of the skin cells that are constantly being shed from humans as well as those of animals and plants etc. This is another factor that binds us with our environment as we take air into the body during inspiration.

Expiration – Breathing Out

- During gaseous exchange, carbon dioxide from the blood is passed into the lungs.
- The diaphragm relaxes into a dome shape.
- The intercostals muscles relax returning the ribs to their normal position
- The thoracic cavity returns to its original shape and the pressure in the lungs increases.
- The lungs recoil to allow the air to flow out of the lungs.

Small amounts of water accompany our outward breath that needs to be replaced to avoid dehydration.

There is a slight pause between the breath in and the breath out whereby the process of gaseous exchange takes place in the lungs. Incoming oxygen is picked up by the blood, transported to the heart to be pumped around the body through arteries.

As the cells of the body receive the oxygen, the carbon dioxide, which has been produced as a result of cellular function, is passed into the blood and transported to the heart through veins, before being received by the lungs to be emitted from the body with the outward breath.

The Art of Breathing

The rate and depth of breathing varies as the body's activity levels change and this process is controlled in the main by the nervous system and involves three types of breathing:

Lateral, costal or normal breathing whereby the lungs take in enough oxygen to accommodate everyday activities as breathing in and out takes place via the nose.

Apical or shallow and rapid breathing whereby the body requires more oxygen during increased physical and mental activity. Mouthfuls of air are taken in and out through the mouth.

Diaphragmatic or deep breathing whereby a controlled intake of breath through the nose is matched with the outward breath either through the nose or mouth.

Poor posture and stress are common causes of poor breathing techniques that impede the natural flow of breath in and out of the body, resulting in physical and mental fatigue.

> Apical breathing accompanies extreme stress resulting in feelings of panic and an inability to catch one's breath. This can be counteracted with some deep diaphragmatic breaths with the emphasis on the outward breath in order to restore body balance and calm the mind.

Water is frequently referred to as a forgotten nutrient. The body's frequent and numerous pleas for it are often ignored, which leads to varying degrees of dehydration and without which life cannot be sustained for more than a few days.

> The human body is made up of approx. two thirds of its own weight in water including:
>
> - Intracellular fluid - the water found in cells with some cells containing as much as 70%
> - Extra cellular fluid - the water that makes up body fluids including blood, sweat and tears, mucus and saliva etc

The Frequent and Numerous Pleas for Water

The body needs a constant supply of water to maintain all its vital functions. Dehydration is accompanied by many symptoms including physical and mental fatigue, loss of concentration, headaches and aching muscles, rapid heartbeat, low blood pressure, indigestion and feelings of nausea, puffiness around the joints, dryness and irritation eg skin, eyes and mouth. Thirst is one of the body's final pleas for hydration and should never be ignored.

> **Water Works:** Try treating all general symptoms associated with 'not feeling quite right' or 'feeling a bit under the weather' with a glass of water in the first instance. You may be surprised at the result.

Fluid Facts

Fluid retention is an often-misunderstood condition and occurs when the body becomes inefficient at releasing excess water. Water, a solvent, acts as a carrier within the body for nutrients and waste products. It also aids in the interchange of nutrients and waste products at a cellular level.

The route of water and waste through the **lymphatic system** is a one way system and relies on movement to aid its flow. Lymphatic vessels run parallel to veins, transporting in the form of fluid lymph the waste the blood is unable to deal with. Fluid retention commonly results in static lymph, which refers to a pooling of fluid in areas such as the ankles where lack of movement has impeded its flow.

Fluid retention occurs if the balance between water input through food and drink and water output through sweat and urine is upset and may be the result of a number of factors including diet, illness, medication, obesity, pregnancy, sedentary lifestyle etc. It often occurs in the lower legs and ankles.

To aid fluid retention in the lower legs and ankles:

- Lie down and raise the legs to a level slightly above the heart

- Massage both the fronts and backs of the lower legs and ankles in an upward direction towards the knee

- Perform gentle ankle and leg exercises throughout the day especially if sitting or standing for long periods

- Wear support tights, stocking or socks. The gentle pressure helps flow

- Avoid a diet high in sugar and salt as these encourage the body to retain water

Medical advice should always be sought if there is any doubt as to the cause of the fluid retention and/or if excessive discomfort or abnormality is experienced.

Oedema refers to the puffiness or swelling associated with fluid retention and may occur anywhere in the body. It may be identified by pressing the affected area with the thumb for two or three seconds – if an indentation remains once the thumb has been released this is a sure sign of oedema.

Fluid retention is common just before and during menstruation when cellulite may be at its worst just before menstruation starts. The varying degrees of oedema are part of the menstrual cycle.

Diuretics encourage the release of fluid in the form of increased urination. They are available in drug or natural form.

Natural diuretics include:

- Teas such as green, dandelion, nettle and fennel

- Cranberry juice

- Apple cider vinegar

> Caffeine is a mild diuretic encouraging increased urine production if drunk in excess. However, caffeine is also a stimulant and it is for this reason that intake should be kept to a minimum.

Dehydration occurs when the bodies need for water is not met and/or the body loses too much water too quickly eg through vomiting and diarrhoea.

As the body's fluid levels drop urine becomes darker in colour and stronger in odour.

Drinking still water at room temperature is the quickest way to restore fluid levels within the body (hydration). Other drinks and watery foods need more processing within the digestive system. The amount of water needed per day is unique to each individual and is dependent on energy production.

> Awareness of the negative effects associated with dehydration and the positive effects of hydration will help a person to determine their own body's pleas for water.

Food is the most easily recognisable of all nutrients and contains the various elements that make up a balanced diet sustaining form and function, and yet life can be maintained for a good few weeks without it.

Nutrients found in food are classified as:

- **Carbohydrates** provide the body with energy. Once digested, they convert into glucose for instant energy and into glycogen for stored energy.

- **Proteins** provide an additional energy source. They are broken down by digestion to form amino acids that are needed by the body primarily for growth and repair as well as for the production of:
  - o enzymes eg the chemicals present in saliva and gastric juices whose function it is to break down food,
  - o hormones ie chemical messengers that instruct the body through its developmental stages,
  - o antibodies that support the body's immune functions,
  - o neurotransmitters that facilitate nerve responses.

- **Fats or lipids** provide a highly concentrated source of energy, which is stored in the body under the skin and called upon whenever carbohydrate intake is reduced or lacking.

- **Vitamins** are organic substances found in many foods that are needed to support the functioning of all of the body systems.

- **Minerals** are inorganic substances mined from the earth that are also needed by the body to support the functioning of the body systems.

- **Fibre** is the largely indigestible parts of plant foods needed by the body to aid ingestion, digestion and excretion.

Metabolism

Metabolism refers to chemical processes - **catabolism** and **anabolism** - that take place in the body whereby substances are converted for use. **Catabolism** refers to the chemical reactions that take place to break down foods into their simplest form for the production of energy and subsequent waste products.

Anabolism refers to the chemical reactions that take place within the body, using energy to produce new parts of a cell structure.

The basal metabolic rate (BMR) refers to the amount of energy required to sustain processes necessary for life. Influenced by many different factors (including age, sex and diet, hormone balance and stress levels) it is measured in calories.

Metabolism Facts

Metabolic rate slows with age

Men have a higher metabolic rate than women

Hormone production affects metabolism

Drinking water aids metabolism

Stress affects metabolism

The body and mind often crave certain foods, which may prove to be at odds with one another, and this is a common cause for eating problems and unnecessary weight gain/loss. The various signs of hunger are often misread whilst others are totally ignored and some even made up as the mind takes over having been guided by the senses.

> The body's need for water is often misread as hunger.

The mind shares strong links with the stomach as:

- The sight, smell, sound, feel and taste of food often lead us to eat more than we need
- Social factors also come into play, which either encourages over or under eating
- Eating habits are formed that are hard to break
- Emotional shifts force changes in eating patterns

A responsible attitude to food together with an understanding of the body's needs is the key to healthy eating. Matching food input with energy output ensures balance and prevents the weight fluctuations that inevitably lead to ill health.

> A little of what you fancy really does do you good feeding both the mind and body. It is when 'a little' becomes 'too much' or 'not enough' that problems arise.

The most intangible and thus under estimated of all the nutrients, **love** nourishes the soul and is responsible for passion, devotion and endearment.

> Learning to love oneself in a non-egotistical way has a knock-on effect on the functioning of cells resulting in greater levels of self respect and self care.

Love for Life

Attitude has a lot to do with personal as well as physical well-being. A positive attitude feeds the cells of the whole body with hope, which has a knock on effect on their development. The opposite is also true.

> There have been numerous occasions where a positive attitude has brought a person back from a near death experience.

Some people believe that the energy of our thoughts produces a vibration that is able to influence the very core of our cells and the phenomenon that may be described as being mind over matter.

Visualisations, affirmations and meditation help a person to tap into this remarkable facility.

> When my father was diagnosed with stomach cancer his chances of survival were minimal. Having been a soldier for much of his working life, he visualised an army coming to his rescue. As the cancer battle raged within his body he planned a counter attack with a military precision that had him visualising his good cells fighting off his bad. Reinforcements came in the form of positive thoughts affirming his defence mechanisms and he managed to live for more years than the medical profession had believed possible.

A positive attitude goes a long way in accepting and respecting the beauty we possess at each stage of our lives and if we believe ourselves to be beautiful we actually encourage others to feel the same.

Light is the ultimate nutrient that binds all of the others together providing the ultimate key to life on earth. Light is the nutrient that links a human being with the strongest force of nature feeding the body, mind and spirit with the energies of the sun and moon. Light contains an array of colours that resonate at differing levels providing a range of subtle energies that have a profound and fortifying effect.

Sunlight is linked with yang energy and moonlight has a yin association. As such, sunlight is energising whilst moonlight has the opposite effect inducing peace and calm. The equilibrium of the body, mind and spirit is reliant on the balance of light, which in turn controls the sleep and wake pattern providing each and every cell with a vital source of nutritional therapy. The pineal gland is a structure within the brain responsible for producing the hormone melatonin in response to fading sunlight preparing the body for sleep. As the body becomes aware of the rising sunlight, melatonin production is halted allowing the body to awaken naturally.

Where There is Light There is Life

Sunlight ensures that life exists on earth through plant photosynthesis.

In addition sunlight has the power to affect humans on a physical, emotional and spiritual level.

When exposed to sunlight the skin produces vitamin D, which is needed in the body to help the bones store calcium. As a result any deficiency in vitamin D leads to weakened bones and problems of the skeletal system. It has also been found that a lack of vitamin D renders the body vulnerable to cancers.

Lack of sunlight is the primary cause of SAD seasonal affective disorder resulting in the 'winter blues'.

Sunlight contains the vibrational energy associated with the colours of the rainbow that form a spiritual connection via the chakras.

The body undergoes a constant need for these collective nutrients, which require fine and intuitive tuning in terms of quantity and quality throughout the natural cycles of life. As a result, not only does each individual cell become a product of that which we breathe, drink and eat as well as how we love and live, so too does each fully formed human being. Beauty therefore is not only dependent on topical care ie what we put onto the body in the form of products, treatments, makeup and perfume etc, but perhaps more so on what we put into it in terms of nutrients.

Fact versus Fad

Nutrients supply us with everything we need on all levels – physical, emotional and spiritual. The key to survival lies in awareness of what, why, when, and how much:

- What nutrients are needed?

- Why nutrients are needed?

- When each nutrient is needed?

- How much of each nutrient is needed?

> Natural light provided early man with a nutritional bonus that is often lacking in the modern world. It is thought that many people today suffer severe sleep deprivation due to the use of electric light. Artificial light has little regard for the rhythms associated with natural light; it forces us to sleep while it is light in the summer and waken while dark in the winter. Although this may suit our lifestyle, it goes against the forces of nature, and many people suffering with SAD as a direct result.

As health and hygiene increased so too did life expectancy and a greater understanding of some of the body's nutritional needs inevitably followed. Treatment of sewage saw the end of many of the life-threatening diseases of the past, and access to clean water became commonplace in the developed world. Travel opened up the trade in food with worldwide import and export widening access and availability and broadening nutritional choices. Refrigeration gave food a longer life span and mass production turned cottage industry food providers, the traditional corner shop and outdoor markets into international manufacturers with indoor mega store supermarkets.

Medical development brought with it the ideology of 'we are what we eat' which led to a greater focus on food nutrition. Conversely, mass production and processing methods, together with synthetic substitution and genetic modification, has imposed increasing nutritional constraints to this ideal.

> The use of pesticides has been linked to cancers, birth defects and fertility problems as well as depression, allergies, migraines and irritable bowel syndrome.

Many medical and nutritional experts now also subscribe to the idea that 'we are what we think' and that our emotions have a direct link with not only with metabolism but also the host of eating disorders and associated health issues that face many people in today's world.

We are what we think. All that we are arises with our thoughts. With our thoughts, we make the world.

Hindu Prince Gautama Siddharta, the founder of Buddhism

> Mental as well as physical stress is a common cause of irritable bowel syndrome – as the body prepares for action it diverts blood away from the digestive organs resulting in a varied set of symptoms depending on the level of the stress and how prolonged it is.

Beauty has always been closely connected to health, and the development of nutritional health within the medical professional saw many parallels within the beauty industry. In the first part of the 20th century the beauty industry took on the role of beautification of the body through nutritional input as well as with products, treatments and exercise. Beauty practitioners began to be comprehensively trained, and beauty therapy qualifications were introduced. Instead of merely selling products, therapists widened their area of expertise and gave hands-on treatment and practical advice that encompassed all these factors.

I remember as a young therapist conducting detailed consultations with clients to include weighing and measuring before providing them with a diet sheet. This would be followed with me putting on my leotard and tights and giving exercise tuition before slipping back into my white uniform to perform a follow up treatment.

As the century progressed and some of these areas developed as specialisms in their own right, with the introduction of clinical nutritionists, personal trainers etc, beauty therapy evolved to such an extent that it now embraces the emotional and spiritual as well as the physical, and offers a truly holistic method of beautification of the body, mind and spirit. As a therapy, the thoughts and feelings surrounding beauty are analysed in as much detail as the processes to achieve beauty are adapted and applied.

Today's therapist will more than likely be qualified in both beauty and holistic therapies and have the ability to adapt her skills to meet the ever-changing and demanding physical, emotional and spiritual needs of the clients she treats – no mean feat!

However, the battle between the external and internal continues to rage, fuelled by a plethora of conflicting nutritional information and advice. We are assailed by myriad macronutrients, micronutrients and antinutrients, free radicals claiming to be death defying, detoxifying and destressing, with the supremacy of the seasonal and super foods to the careful combining and colour coordination of our groceries. Is this distracting us from the basic reality of the body's need for nourishment?

Glossary of Terms

- **Macronutrients:** nutrients needed in bulk by the body including water, carbohydrates, proteins and fats. Love and light may be classified as being macronutrients.

- **Micronutrients:** nutrients needed in minute quantities by the body, including vitamins and minerals.

- **Antinutrients:** anything that stops the nutritious benefit of a nutrient eg cigarettes, alcohol, pesticides etc.

- **Free radicals:** the by-product of energy production, responsible for the ageing process. Internally free radicals are produced as a result of cellular activity. External examples include pollution.

- **Death defying, detoxifying and destressing foods:** nutrients that fight free radical attack to delay the ageing process eg vitamins A, C and E, nutrients that stimulate the removal of cellular waste eg water and nutrients with a calming effect eg alkaline foods.

- **Seasonal and superfoods:** it is argued that eating seasonal foods maintains harmony between the earth and its inhabitants through the rhythms of nature whilst superfoods is a term given to food with high phytonutrient content ie chemical compounds that occur naturally in plants eg beta-carotene and provide exceptional nutrition and medicinal properties

- **Food combining and colour coordination:** from the potentially balancing effect of certain nutrients and neutralising effect of the natural colour of food resulting in maximum nutritional value for holistic wellbeing.

Can Beauty Be Achieved by Taking a Pill or Applying a Potion?

If we subscribe to the notion that 'we are what we eat' it may be realistic to expect that beauty can indeed be achieved through the nutrients we put into our bodies.

However, the problems lie in our expectations of beauty, which are too often unrealistic and as such, unattainable. Having an awareness of our inherent body type, ie ectomorph, mesomorph and endomorph, helps us understand the workings of the body and how it is able to gain and lose weight. These inherited characteristics mean that we are unable to make drastic changes to our body shape without the intervention of surgery.

Ectomorphs do not gain weight easily and are more likely to be long and lean in figure.

Mesomorphs gain weight slowly and are more likely to be muscular and curvaceous in figure.

Endomorphs gain weight easily and are more likely to be rounded in figure.

Knowledge of our inherent tendencies helps in the acceptance of our physical limitations.

You don't have to look very far to find a diet designed to achieve every aspect of beauty known to man and indeed woman kind. From busting fat to calming karma there are as many diets that claim to enhance inner beauty, as there are those for outer beauty. But there is not much we can to do alter our basic body shape and tendencies.

There is also the idea that beauty may be achieved through supplements and remedies.

Supplements are products that contain one or more of a person's dietary needs and seek to help the body to maintain its functions and/or repair those affected by deficiency.

Remedies are seen as being more medicinal in their action.

Both supplements and remedies have a supporting role and should not be seen as replacements for nutrients.

Supplements and remedies can:

- Aid a specific nutrient deficiency
- Boost the nutritional value of a diet
- Reduce for some the risk of certain disorders
- Support health at the different stages of the life cycle
- Help to restore health and build immunity post illness and/or surgery
- Assist in balancing moods, feelings and emotions

They can't always provide a quick fix, nor are they always successful.

Their origins and toxicity are not always clear.

Put into context therefore, beauty comes from good health, which comes from good nutrition, which may be enhanced by the supportive nature and correct use of supplements and remedies, but it must also be remembered that nutrition does not refer to food alone. Oxygen, water, love and light are just as important.

Beauty is therefore the whole deal and as such, is more than just the sum of the parts.

CHAPTER SIX

Sound

Seeing, hearing and feeling are miracles,
and each part and tag of me is a miracle.
Walt Whitman

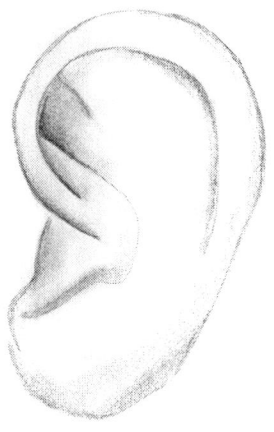

The Science of Sound

The frequencies associated with sound waves are carried by the surrounding air and enter the body through the opening of the ears. The eighth cranial nerves known as the **vestibulocochlear** nerves carry the frequencies to the **temporal lobes** of the brain where sound information is analysed by the **auditory cortex**.

The different frequencies are split up, then analysed as this part of the brain recognises and identifies what the sound is and where it came from. Speech is analysed mostly by the left temporal lobes of the brain and music mostly by the right.

This function facilitates the recognition of another layer of beauty – that which is associated with not only the beauty of the sound itself but also of the sentiment behind the sound.

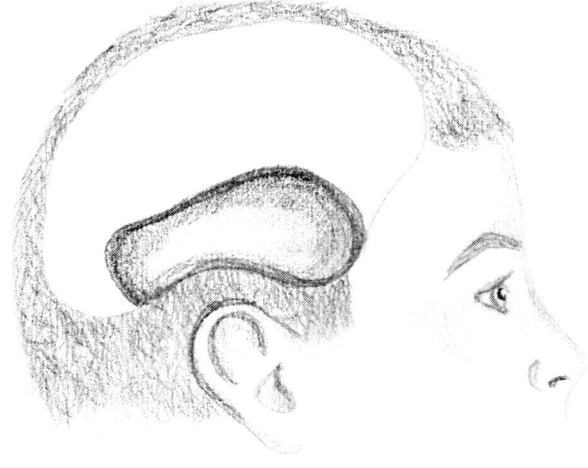

SENSE OF SOUND

The Art of Sound

Clairaudience, clear hearing, often linked with clairvoyance is another of the extra sensory functions and refers to the hearing of sounds that are not normally physically audible by humans and is believed to be associated with hearing the vibrations or vibes from the past and even the future.

The ears are believed to have heavenly, human and earthly links through their upper, middle and lower parts. Since the ear is the only facial feature that does not move, some say that it cannot lie, and therefore its structure portrays a person's true self.

As with the eyes and iridology, the ears also contain an image of the body as a whole, which may be treated through the stimulation of reflex points and a treatment known as **ear reflexology**. Developed in the west in the 1950s ear reflexology has had an even longer association with the Chinese tradition of acupuncture aiming to treat each part of the body through the treatment of specific points on the ear. A map of the body may be viewed as an image of an inverted foetus is transposed onto the ear.

Gentle manipulation of each point may be carried out using the fingers and/or a small tool to bring about a sense of physical, emotional and spiritual balance in much the same way as the more widely recognised treatment of hand or foot reflexology.

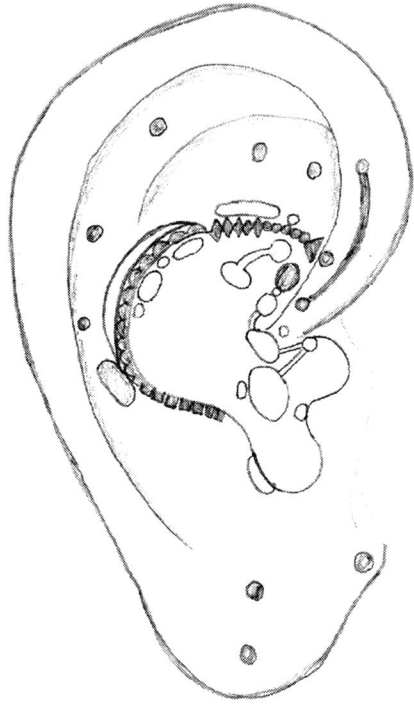

EAR REFLEX POINTS

Ear Facts – The Physical Ear

The external portion of the ear or earflap is known as the **auricle** or **pinna** and is divided into the **upper helix** and **lower lobule** or **lobe**. The helix is made from fibro cartilage and as such is firmer in structure and has a poor blood supply, whilst the lobe is fleshier, more flexible and rich in blood.

The inner portion of the external ear is known as the **concha**, taking its name from its shell-like form. Several muscles attach to the ear but they remain undeveloped.

The **auditory canal** forms an s-shaped tube leading into the eardrum. Fine hairs line the skin of the auditory canal together with glands responsible for the formation of **cerumen** (ear wax) both of which offer a form of protection against particles entering deep into the ear.

The **ear drum** or **tympanic membrane** is cone-shaped, consisting of an outer covering of hairless skin, a middle layer of fibrous tissue and an inner lining of mucous membrane.

Beyond the eardrum lies an irregular-shaped cavity known as the **middle ear** containing three small bones, which form a bridge between the eardrum and the inner ear. The inner ear consists of fluid filled tubes or labyrinths which form semicircular canals and are responsible for maintaining a sense of physical balance, together with the **cochlea**, which is responsible for the sensory function associated with hearing.

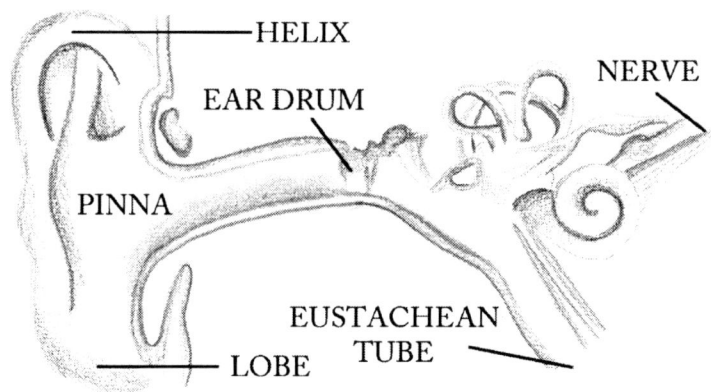

Ear Facts – The Emotional Ear

Sound can cause emotional changes within the body; voice is the most primitive and powerful means to express feeling. Music provides another emotional stimulus, arousing a host of emotions depending on personal interpretation and may be used to sedate or stimulate as we are intuitively drawn to listen to the genre of music that appeals to our emotional needs at any time. The combination of voice and music creates a full circle of therapy allowing emotions into and out of the body with the accompanying sounds. Beauty as an emotion may be experienced and acknowledged through sound.

The sound of the conscience may also be heard. This method of hearing subscribes to the idea of an inner voice associated with reason and emotional truth.

Ear facts - The Spiritual Ear

It is believed that there exists a third ear that hears and responds to sound at a higher and more spiritual level via the seven main **chakras**. At this level, each chakra responds specifically to a musical note thus strengthening and balancing its associated energy, function and spiritual links eg

- A – sixth: brow chakra
- B – seventh: crown chakra
- C – first: base chakra
- D – second: sacral chakra

- E – third solar: plexus chakra
- F – fourth: heart chakra
- G – fifth: throat chakra

Sound is a form of energy that vibrates at different levels in much the same way as individual cells of the body, mind and spirit vibrate as they produce the energy needed to perform their specific functions.

Sound affects physical, emotional and spiritual changes. Sound therapy describes the use of musical notes to balance energy at a cellular level, which in turn has a far-reaching effect in creating a greater sense of wellbeing. A sound therapist will use a mixture of individual musical notes to affect specific changes in a quest for overall balance and harmony.

By tapping into the physical, emotional and spiritual ears, there exists the means for a deeper truth to be heard with the potential to question or confirm first impressions of beauty.

Ear Beauty

The ears should be shell-like in shape, firm yet flexible in texture, small and neat.

According to the rules of symmetry, the perfect ear should be set on a level between the eyebrow and the tip of the nose within the middle third of the head. Both ears should be in line with each other, lie close to the head, be of a smooth and even shape with fleshy lobes.

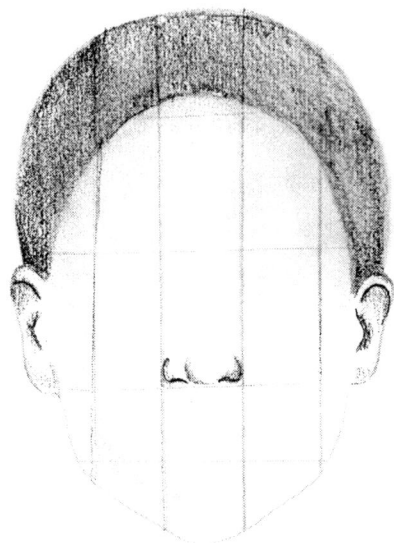

THE PERFECT EAR

It is believed that people with very prominent ears may have experienced some form of foetal distress.

Unlike the eyes or the skin, the ears are not naturally beautiful and do not score highly in the first impressions associated with physical attractiveness.

Any defects in the perfect shape, size and position may be covered by a clever hairstyle whilst perfection may be further enhanced by the age-old tradition of ear piercing. Piercing of the external portion of the ear is a universal practice for both men and women and one where the creative, fashionable and individual styles of beauty can be expressed. The ear is not only the most popular part of the body to be pierced but also the easiest; the earlobe is bone and cartilage free and as a result quick to heal.

Beautiful woods, metals and stones have been to be used to decorate and draw attention to the human body as well as display the wealth and status of an individual. For many traditions the ears are seen as pathways into the heart and the items used to adorn the ear lobes used to ward off possible invaders of the body as well boost its beauty and attractiveness.

Ear Piercing Rituals

Ritual ear stretching or gauging has been used by some cultures as a rite of passage from childhood into puberty and is a procedure that has been adopted in more modern times by those wishing to progress their piercings.

A hole is made in the earlobe as with a regular piercing and allowed to heal. The hole is then stretched and a variety of different sized rings are inserted and regularly changed in order to gradually increase the stretch.

There is a point of no return – the point where the hole will no longer close up and heal over if left free of the ring. Depending on the individual elasticity of the skin, this is approx 10 – 15mm.

The upper helix and inner flap of the ear may also be pierced but as these areas have a large cartilage content which does not receive such a good blood supply as the fleshier lobe, they do not readily heal. This has not stopped them from being very popular piercing sites but remain slightly less socially acceptable along with the stretching methods in today's culture.

Ear Power

It is claimed to be possible through focused thought and meditation to increase the power of the ears to such an extent that they are able to pick up the ultra, infra and cosmic levels of sound. There is a belief amongst some that all particles on earth and beyond emit varying amounts of frequencies or sound vibrations, most of which the human ear is unable to detect.

The sound of silence associated with a meditative state is thought to stimulate the so-called third ear and evoke some of these sounds. **Thermal auricular therapy** commonly referred to as ear candling is a treatment traditionally used by native Indian tribes as a means of preparation for such a state. Introduced into the west in recent years it is primarily used to clear the ears on a physical level but users are also conscious of the very real benefits the treatment has on bringing about a sense of peace and calm and in doing so creating a greater sense of spiritual awareness.

The candles used in thermal auricular therapy bear no resemblance to wax candles other than the fact that they are lit. Generally comprised of a rolled tube or cone of flax in which active ingredients such as propolis and St John's Wort are held in the base, the candles are placed at the opening of the ear and the top is lit. As it burns, it creates a chimney effect gently drawing excess moisture, warming the surrounding area, stimulating blood and lymphatic flow and creating a soothing and healing effect as the active ingredients get to work.

The Language of the Ear

It is possible to listen without hearing and vice versa as a person tunes in or out of the sounds around them. 'Falling on deaf ears' refers to just this – the ears have heard but the mind has failed to engage. This falls into the category of sensory adaptation, which allows for familiar sounds to be ignored and contributes to the idea of selective hearing. In addition, failing to make use of or wrongly interpreting body language will render a person incapable of interpreting the sentiments behind the spoken word.

Without the ability to hear, speech becomes very difficult. In order to allow for the replication of sound the mind ideally needs to have heard it first. Whilst a deaf person can copy the tongue and mouth movements that shape the outgoing air to form a coherent sound the resulting noise is often a poor imitation of the original.

Ear Care

As part of the special senses, the ears require special care to maintain their functions associated with balance and hearing as well as help to contribute to the impressions of beauty.

Water intake contributes to the formation of cerumen (ear wax), which is produced in the auditory canal as a means of protection for the inner workings of the ear.

Waterworks: The ears are linked to the back of the nose via the Eustachian tube, which is prone to congestion in both directions contributing to the pressure levels within the head. Gulping a mouthful of water not only hydrates but also helps to open the Eustachian tube releasing and equalising the pressure resulting in clearing the links between the ears, nose and throat.

Resting the ears is vital for their well-being not only through the power of sleep. Times of quiet in a daily routine enables the ears to become more attuned to the world around them.

The sense of hearing is diminished greatly when the ears are subjected to excessive amounts of loud sounds. Sound is measured in decibels (dB). A whisper measures approximately 40dB and normal conversation approximately 65dB.

The sound levels produced at a concert can reach up to 120dB and may result in acoustical trauma – pain, discomfort and even damage to the middle and inner ear.

Ear checks and hearing tests ensure the wellbeing of the ear which is monitored and any defects detected and treated. Hearing problems may be the result of many factors, which may prove severe in the long term if not caught early.

Loss of hearing may be classified as being conductive or sensorineural:

Conductive - sound transmission abnormalities present in the middle or outer ear that can usually be corrected.

Sensorineural - involves the workings within the inner ear and is much more difficult to treat.

Monitoring the ears can help to lessen and/or avoid such problems.

The ears should be cleaned with care and any excess earwax removed with caution. They are, for the most part, self-cleaning. The tiny hairs lining the auditory canal together with the production of earwax trap and prevent particles of dirt and dust from entering. Jaw movements made during eating, drinking and talking serve to gently ease the earwax to the outer portion of the ears. Cotton buds are often used, but they push earwax further into the ear and cause damage and pain if inserted too far. A tissue used to gently wipe the entrance to the auditory canal is a much safer option.

> Nothing smaller than the width of a finger should be inserted into the ear for fear of possible damage.

Because of their links with the nose and throat via the Eustachian tube, the ears are susceptible to the following:

- Extreme discomfort if the Eustachian tube becomes blocked as pressure builds to create a vacuum in the middle ear. This forces the eardrum inwards and stretches it painfully taut

- Infection from the nose and/or throat transferred to the ears and vice versa

- Loss or impaired hearing caused by congestion, trauma or damage

Special Care

Splashing the face with water in an upward direction prior to blowing the nose at the end of the day will clear the passageways between the nose and the ears helping to clear congestion and prevent infection.

Yawning and swallowing both help to release pressure build up having an equalising effect on the ears.

Avoiding excess intake of salt, caffeine, tobacco and dairy foods, which are all known triggers for ear problems.

Checking the side effects of drugs taken for medicinal purposes, many of which can result in unwanted symptoms associated with the ears.

Keeping the ears dry, warm and draught free maintains comfort and wellbeing.

Ear massage provides a multi-functional aid, is easy to apply and can be carried out as required:

Gentle massage movements to the ears and pressure points in the surrounding area stimulates blood flow, drains lymph, eases congestion and soothes irritation

A gentle pull around the edges of the ears helps to unblock the Eustachian tubes

Cupping the hand over the ears for a few moments calms and warms the ears

Gentle massage manipulations over the whole ear aid the reflex points associated with the rest of the body

> Ear massage is a great self help tool, takes but a moment and can have an holistic effect on wellbeing

The emotional ear needs to be finely tuned if it is to pick up the subtleties of the spoken word. Hearing the meaning behind the sounds relies on a clear and open mind and one of the best ways of achieving this is to practice silent meditation.

> Listening to the sound of silence can be a challenge as the inner voice takes over with a barrage of thoughts and feelings. Acknowledging them but allowing them to pass is the surest way to silence the mind.

The spiritual third ear also benefits from special care helping to keep the channels of energy clear so that sounds become more audible at all levels.

> **Spiritual Care:** Affirmations offer a positive voice of intent and may take on the form of an internal or external sound. Internally affirmations may be linked with positive thinking whilst externally a word or phrase often referred to as a mantra can be said or sung out loud. *Om* is widely recognised as a universal mantra with far reaching effects.

Hearsay

Prior to the 20th century beauty boom in mass production the commercial world was a very different place from the one we inhabit today. Knowledge and resources were not only limited but also restricted to regions and travel was painfully slow and fraught with dangers. Lack of education meant that many people were unable to read and write and so word of mouth remained the only sure means of communication.

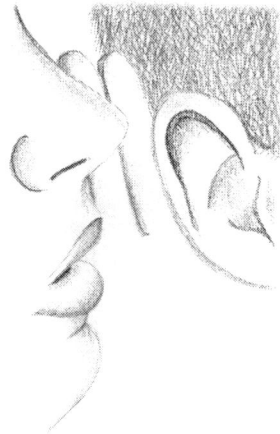

HEARSAY

Early beauty entrepreneurs peddled their wares gypsy-style from village to village, town to town, city to city and region to region, attending fetes and fairs. There were plenty of bogus products claiming to be 'beauty in bottle' or 'cure alls'. Like the travelling vendors of today who illegally set up on street corners with their suitcases, these peddlers made sure that they left well before their claims could be refuted or questioned.

> All truths begin with hearsay.

The door-to-door method of selling followed, with many companies making their debuts in this way.

> Avon was originally known as The California Perfume Company and was founded in 1886 by a door-to-door salesman. The name was changed in 1939 and Avon was introduced into Britain in 1959. Avon remains a popular door-to-door product company albeit updated to meet today's market with the introduction of internet shopping.

As the economy developed and shops and businesses became more established, creative signage and window displays alerted the illiterate to the products and services on sale within.

> The distinctive red and white barber's shop sign has stood the test of time.

Whilst the 18th and 19th centuries saw developments in science and medicine, healthcare was still by and large associated more with luck than judgment and beauty a luxury afforded by the wealthy.

Lack of nutrition and poor sanitary conditions for all but the upper classes made beauty short-lived. Life expectancy was significantly lower than it is now and people could spend little or no time on the care and beautification of the body.

Women's historically inferior place in society together with a lack of birth control and medical care took its toll as physical and emotional wear and tear from multiple pregnancies, frequent infant death as well as a high probability of their own death in childbirth were commonplace.

Men also paid a high physical and emotional price as brutal wars were fought often by hand. Malnutrition, disfigurement and loss of limbs as well as life accompanied such times. Disease was rife and almost impossible to control within the poor living conditions.

There was little time or possibility to concentrate on maintaining physical beauty.

However, as the western world progressed, so too did the health and wealth of its people which inevitably had an effect on their beauty aspirations. Life took on a different meaning as education, medical care, opportunities for work and safer living conditions became available.

Economic change took place with the development of new technology and the subsequent mass production led to lifestyle changes. Greater access to education went hand in hand with the introduction and progression of publicised information at the start of the 20th century, which in turn led to a word revolution.

New channels of communication opened up which coincided with the development of health products and procedures, and culminated with a beauty boom that shows no signs of losing pace. The universal printed word, telephones, radio, film and television made health and beauty information and advertising increasingly accessible and with the advent of the Internet ever more so.

Print reinforced the spoken voice, the educated access to great minds, and medical studies raised health levels. Newspapers, periodicals and magazines encouraged companies to inform the public of their wares and a shopping culture developed that was further enhanced by the introduction of mail order. As earnings increased, so too did access to affordable products.

Rimmel was amongst many of the up and coming companies who sold their products through mail order. Rimmel also made use of the programmes of London's theatres to inform the type of people they hoped to attract of the benefits of their products.

Yardley and Innoxa sent out free booklets by request from their Bond Street salons. Yardley's was entitled 'Secrets from Bond Street' whilst Innoxa offered 'the truest, most exciting, most romantic book on beauty ever written.'

During the war years, women's magazines printed helpful make-do-and-mend makeup hints eg 'scrape out and melt down the base of old lipsticks to create a new shade'.

From black and white silent movies to talkies and eventually Technicolor, fashion met with beauty on the big screen to form a powerful creative force that was to be felt across the world.

Classical European cities such as Paris and London were a perfect match for the glamour of Hollywood and the fast moving innovations of America's technology. Movie stars became the global symbols of modern health and beauty whilst the glamorous beauty entrepreneurs became its voice. In no time, the resulting images of beauty and the products that were claimed to produce them acquired a cult status around the world. Health care became a necessity of life and cosmetics its acceptable enhancement.

> **Movie Madness:** Movie stars have showcased the fashion and beauty of each era with product companies evolving to meet their demands.
>
> Beauty styles have yo-yoed between upfront sexuality, the mysterious and androgynous, glamour and wholesome femininity, and the beauty industry has adapted its products to appeal to every woman and ensure she has had access to the means to recreate those on-screen images for herself.

Radio and eventually television brought the sound of beauty into the home with sponsorship and advertising, and the introduction of colour TV fuelled the desire to recreate the more realistic images of beauty seen on the small screen. The music industry with its pop videos and pop idols and the fashion industry with its catwalk shows and super models introduced a younger audience of both sexes to the many and varied faces of beauty that was beginning to emerge. The links between the arts were firmly grounded in beauty with the media cementing the bonds.

> Colour TV was launched in America in the mid 1950s, and in Europe in the 1960s. However it wasn't until the 70s that most households had one. Twenty-four hour airtime and multiple channels followed as new technology leads the way for consumer demands.

As the fantasy and glamour of film gave way to reality television the Celebrity Culture of recent years has emerged, fuelled by the paparazzi who are on hand to record the good, the bad and the ugly faces of beauty. With every beauty genre fast becoming the focus of intense scrutiny, the high gloss and full definition photographs of the fashion magazines have all but replaced the illustrations of the past periodicals.

This in turn has led to a pendulum of beauty which swings between photo manipulation fantasy and warts and all reality communicating a set of mind-muddling, mixed messages.

Celebrity endorsement has seen word of mouth communication reach an all time high providing an enviable additional source of income for the celebrities, a high profile platform for product companies and a must have culture that the consumer is unable to ignore. By the same token, the desire to see the very same celebrities fall from grace is ever present.

The Internet and connected technology has opened up channels of communication all over the world at any time of the day or night. At the click of a button we can connect, view and review to our heart's content. We can fast forward or rewind to make changes to our here and now.

A virtual world has been created in which we are able to follow beauty fashion and trend without moving, look at what's new without being seen, listen to the hype without being noticed and even update our status and create an interactive voice without making a sound and as we spend without handing over any cash, we are all but finding beauty without even thinking.

Beauty has emerged as one of the most media-ridden and controversial commodities of the modern world and may be held accountable for a lot of what is bad as well as good in today's commercial culture.

Tried and Tested

The massive influx of health, beauty and eventually makeup products in the 20th century, together with the advances made in medical and health care, mean that control is needed more than ever before. Mass production meant mass usage and moves were made to ensure that mass abuse did not automatically follow.

In America the Federal Food, Drug and Cosmetic Act FDA was introduced in 1938, which was closely followed by British Cosmetic Regulations and European laws that ensure the safety of products used for the health and beautification of the body.

Cosmetics refer to all retail and professional products that can be rubbed, poured, sprinkled or sprayed onto the body in order to enhance its appearance or smell and include:

- Cleansers, toners, creams, balms, oils and gels
- Makeup
- Shampoos, conditioners and hair dyes
- Hygiene products
- Fragrances
- All products are assessed for:
- Ingredients, composition and testing
- Packaging and labeling
- Storage and shelf life

The flood of health, beauty and makeup products also brought with it the opportunity of the development of new as well as old skills. The art of dressing hair, the creative application of makeup and the treatment of the face and body for care and beautification which had once been the domain of the ladies maid emerged as a career route for aspiring men as well as women. Hair and beauty salons were opened in the fashion and style centres of the world notably Paris, New York and London where beauty and fashion forged strong links which added to their influence and kudos as stand alone industries.

Just as the products themselves needed regulating so did their usage and application. The development of treatment procedures necessitated training, which needed to be monitored. Schools dedicated to beauty training were introduced along with qualifications that specified treatment standards. Codes of practice and ethics were introduced to uphold the respectability that the beauty industry was cultivating, and to raise its profile.

What started as a small cottage style trade with a few players is now a multi billion pound industry that commands attention at all levels.

Education is ensuring that practitioners maintain the same standards as all other professionals. The health, beauty and cosmetic industry in the 21st century is divided into separate units each with its own transferable skills and qualifications at all levels of the educational spectrum, with access to study starting as young as 14, with no upper age limit. Beauty has become a job for life and a career for many.

Qualified practitioners were encouraged to insure themselves and their practices in an attempt to further safeguard the general public against product abuse and treatment misadventure.

Show and sell trade fairs and exhibitions provided manufacturers with a platform from which to communicate beauty innovations to practitioners. Magazines dedicated to the beauty industry offered an additional source of information as did the publication of technical books and learning resources. By the time I entered the industry in the 1970s beauty was firmly on the commercial map of the world, shrugging off its questionable past and growing in credibility with every new product innovation and accompanying buzzword.

Fact or Fiction

- The power of words to create what we want to hear
- The power of an image to recreate what we want to see
- The power of advertising to make us want to buy, buy and then buy some more

The beauty industry has created an interconnected cycle of mass production and mass media within which legislation has gone a long way to safeguard consumer rights: from product safety to discrimination and sexual equality, from treatment liability, to sale of goods and data protection.

Advertising, like beauty, touches and stimulates each of our senses and sometimes all sense of reason disappears as perception takes over. Effective advertising follows four key stages including attention, perception, association and memory.

1. First impressions associated with the sight, feel, sound, smell and/or taste of a product are designed to create an initial impact that has the power to grab the attention of the consumer literally stopping them in their tracks.

> The more senses stimulated, the more powerful the impact. The sales girls and boys who walk around the department stores with a perfume bottle in their hands aim to tap into all of our senses – eyes feast on the beauty of the sales person, skin feels the seductive spray of the perfume, olfaction occurs as the fragrance is breathed in and the taste buds are stimulated with the outward breath.

2. The brain interprets the sensations and makes an instant decision as to the perceived personal benefits of the product resulting in the 'I like it /I like it not' response.

> Through meticulous marketing, advertisers get into the mindset of their target audience, which serves to anticipate a positive reaction.

3. An 'I like it' response will be followed up with some justifying action that enables the consumer to make a direct association with the product resulting in an 'I need/want it' response.

> A secondary impact is created that provides a special personal message that is difficult to ignore eg special benefits, special offer or special price.

4. This information is either acted upon immediately and/or stored in the consumer's memory bank for future use.

> The final impact is something that binds the consumer to the product eg a tagline or motto and which serves to encourage brand loyalty.

Trial and error accompanied the early advertisements for skin care, which were in black and white and usually featured the benefits of the product more than the product itself. Scare tactics often accompanied the advertisements for anti ageing products inferring the damage that may result if a certain product is NOT used. Many of the early product companies made celebrity claims. For instance, Ponds declared that 'countless thousands of women including 82 famous actresses' used their creams!

Targets in the early days of beauty advertising:

- **Women of all social classes:** mass production meant that there were suitable products available for everyone and advertising provided the means to reach all levels of society.

- **Older women wishing to appear younger:** as mature women began to take more of an active role in society, they were encouraged to look their best through the advertising of specific anti aging products.

- **Younger women wishing to appear more glamorous:** through celebrity endorsements advertisers ensured that certain products gained a cult following.

- **Working women:** women began to compete in a male-dominated world. Advertisers advocated good grooming as a means to empowerment. During the war years Yardley's advertisements talked about women's war jobs and the need to 'put your best face forward' by using their complexion powder.

- **Women in search of a husband:** advertisements that offered romantic solutions to catching a man ensured the sale of many products. Advertisements frequently featured either the femme fatale or the femme fragile images in a bid to provide a broad appeal and to demonstrate the growing product choices available to women in search of romance.

The only beauty advertisements that were aimed at men were associated with the sale of perfumes, which were almost exclusively purchased by men and as such were often sultry and seductive.

> Popular perfumes during the first part of the 20th century:
>
> - Dans La Nuit (In The Night) 1924
> - Vers le Jour (Just Before Dawn) 1925
> - Sans Adieu (Because I Can't Bear to Say Goodbye) 1929
> - Je Reviens (I Will Return) 1932
> - Vers Toi (To You) 1934

Men did not feature in beauty advertising until the second half of the 20th century when men's grooming began to take on a focus of its own. Advertisements tended to be one-dimensional, with macho images that portrayed the strength and virility of men through masculine ideals and endorsements eg the nautical theme of Old Spice and the sportsmen who endorsed Faberge's Brut.

The postwar beauty boom saw product manufacture become more sophisticated, and also methods of advertising. Fierce competition led to companies developing their unique selling points (USPs) in order to outdo their rivals. Makeup gained more focus and advertisers were able to achieve greater levels of success by the use of a varied colour palette and highly descriptive product names.

> Product Names veered between shy and shocking. In the shy corner lipsticks and nail enamels had names that were preceded by soft references with innocent and virginal feminine images
>
> - Heavenly peach
> - Ballet pink
> - Almost apricot

> In the shocking corner strong references were made with the use of names with darker, sexier undertones that carried the promise of seduction and empowerment
>
> - Captivating coral
> - Dynamite red
> - Torrid peach

Colour and choice was the order of 1960s beauty, with advertising setting the scene. Product companies extended their ranges and demand rocketed, with the new youth culture that saw Mary Quant not only change the face of fashion but also that of beauty.

> Advertisements for Mary Quant makeup described 'the makeup that looks like it isn't there' heralding the start of the natural look for faces. The advertisements also boasted that the makeup range contained 26 different shades of nail enamels and 26 of lipsticks.

As the second half of the 20th century got firmly under way, women became more financially independent and wanted to look good for themselves rather than just to catch a man.

Skin care, makeup and perfume became an integral part of most women's lifestyles and product companies made sure that there was ample choice to suit everyone's pocket. The advertising companies thought up new and exciting campaigns that had all age groups from teenagers to octogenarians clamouring for the latest product 'to die for'. Designer labels made their way on to packaging and even carrier bags as products gained in eye appeal, kudos and the wow factor.

> Clever advertising has seen the consumer become a walking advertisement every time they make a purchase and carry the logo bearing carrier bag for all to see.

'Limited Edition' has accelerated impulse buying and if you are not on the latest waiting lists for 'newest formula product' you are out of the loop. Through advertising, products have been able to communicate powerful messages that have not only got under the skin of the consumer but have infiltrated the Id and appealed to the ego so much so that it is impossible to differentiate between products we actually need and those we simply desire. Any justification to purchase, if we need it, is just a tag line or scientific claim away and if that is not enough, reassurance may be found because after all *you are worth it.*

Iconic Beauty Products

Mary Quant's white lipstick changed the face of a generation and will be forever associated with the look of the 60s.

Rouge Noir nail enamel was first seen on the Chanel catwalk in 1994. This never seen before blend of red and black developed cult status becoming Chanel's best selling product and prompting a host of copycat enamels by other brands

Cacharel's Anais Anais captured the hearts of a generation of women with its soft feminine fragrance. Named after the goddess of fertility Anaitis and launched in 1979, it became iconic of the era.

> Bourjois little round pots of blusher and eye shadow have been around since 1863. The original products were produced using a revolutionary baking technique. Today, these iconic products have been updated and contain 80% mineral pigments.
>
> It is reported that one pot of Elizabeth Arden's Eight Hour Cream is sold every minute in the UK. What began as a salve to soothe the skin of her race horses developed into one of the must have products of our time.

Innovation and temptation became the name of the selling game, with advertising campaigns selling hard through methods fair or foul. Verbal trickery, image manipulation and the constant bombardment of the senses encourages 21st-century consumers to buy with their ethereal rather than with their common sense.

> The language of cosmetics has become a blend of technology and creation resulting in techno talk, buzz words and jargon. Technical terms adding kudos to everyday words eg the use of Derma for skin, amino acids for proteins
>
> An unrealistic beauty ideal is often presented with youthful models advertising anti-ageing brands and the use of enhanced images eg hair and lash extensions
>
> Clever use of *before and after* images (usually unsmiling before and smiley after) compounding the belief of an ugly past and a beautiful future
>
> Sophisticated packaging projecting the temptation of the beauty held within that many are unable to resist
>
> A *try me* culture encouraging consumers to *stop, try and buy*

Throughout the years product companies have been bought and sold, amalgamated and homogenised in the name of progress. Beauty has grown up and become big business, and like all businesses it needs to do some active listening in order to hear the future.

Beauty is as beauty does.

Epilogue

All we have to believe with is our senses, the tools we use to perceive the world: our sight, our touch, our memory. if they lie to us, then nothing can be trusted. And even if we do not believe, then still we cannot travel in any other way then the road our senses show us; and we must walk that road to the end.

Neil Galman

A Phenomenon of Extremes

At the shallow end, beauty occurs when the senses fail to fully engage with the brain, resulting in a one-dimensional form of perception. It is fickle, fashionable and fun offering a quick fix, and may be described as being beauty without the use of sensible senses.

For some, this form of beauty is artificial and expressionless and senseless, sharing its associations with vanity and ego.

At the deep end, beauty occurs when the brain engages with the senses to reach perception at a multi-dimensional level. It is has a conscience, is knowledgeable and questioning and may be described as being beauty with a soul.

Some see this form of beauty as natural and organic, sharing its associations with the Id and the psyche.

The law of opposites and the concept of *yin* and *yang* state that you cannot have one extreme without the other. Perhaps herein lies the key to beauty.

Most people will spend a lifetime yo-yoing between the two extremes with either a mindless or mindful view of the associated influences and pressures.

A mindless view sees us at either end of the beauty spectrum without being aware of how or why we got there resulting in a beauty mismatch as the physical and spiritual parts of a person become out of synch.

A view that is mindful, on the other hand, will find some of us as happy at the shallow end of beauty with our feet as firmly on the ground as those others at the deeper end going with the flow.

Ultimately, the true essence of beauty will be found as a person settles somewhere within the two beauty extremes in a place that sees them comfortable, accepted and loved.

Beauty is truth, truth beauty

John Keats

About The Author

Tina Parsons is founder and
principal of the multi award
winning Burghley Academy
training school and salon as
well as an experienced teacher
of beauty and holistic therapies.
Tina is a popular author of a
range of leading text books and
is dedicated to developing
standards within the industry.

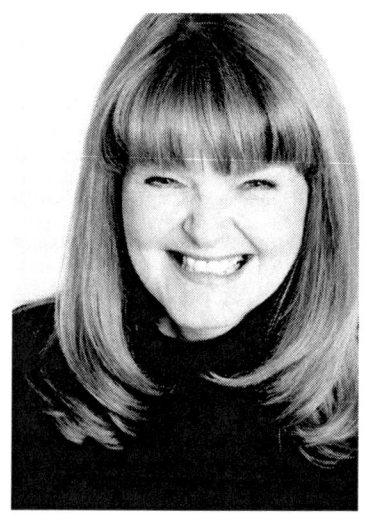

Burghley academy

Burghley Academy is a family owned business founded in 1981 that incorporates hairdressing, beauty and holistic therapies within an impressive 15ᵗʰ century building in the heart of the Cathedral City of Peterborough. Run by Tina, her husband Chris and more recently their daughter Alexa, Burghley Academy Training was established in 1989 and has become a leading private training school in the midlands attracting students from across the UK, and has over the years won a host of local and national business, therapy and training awards. We believe:

- In lifelong learning
- If you want to move mountains. start by moving little stones
- The world steps aside when you know exactly where you are going
- People show what they are by what they do with what they have
- Inspiration is an energy just waiting to be used
- We should listen with our heads and go with our hearts
- Some dream of doing great things, others stay awake and do them
- We should live what we learn
- The most important things in life aren't things

www.burghleyacademy.org

Lightning Source UK Ltd.
Milton Keynes UK
UKOW021511301111

182944UK00003B/4/P